The Fertile Years

By the same author

No Change: A Biological Revolution for Women

Wendy Cooper

The Fertile Years

Hutchinson of London

Acknowledgement

The Fertile Years could never have been written without the encouragement and patient help of many doctors, and I can only hope they will accept that occasional criticisms apply not to the individual doctor so much as to the system, of which they can be the victim just as much as the patient.

Hutchinson & Co. (Publishers) Ltd
3 Fitzroy Square, London W I P 6JD

London Melbourne Sydney Auckland
Wellington Johannesburg and agencies
throughout the world

First published 1978
© Wendy Cooper 1978

Set in Monotype Baskerville

Printed in Great Britain by The Anchor Press Ltd
and bound by Wm Brendon & Son Ltd
both of Tiptree, Essex

ISBN 0 09 136120 6

Contents

Foreword

by Professor Stuart Campbell, FRCOG,
Department of Obstetrics and Gynaecology,
King's College Hospital Medical School

The past twenty-five years have witnessed a remarkable expansion of medical knowledge, especially in the area of health care for women. These advances have also resulted in a social revolution for women such as no politician could hope to achieve in several lifetimes. The poverty trap of the 1930s, when women were doomed to have one unwanted pregnancy after another, has been eliminated by efficient contraceptive techniques, and by early and safe abortion. Pregnancy and labour is now a much safer and happier experience for both mother and baby, and the chances of the infertile couple being helped toward having their own child are now better than ever before.

British obstetricians and gynaecologists have been foremost in bringing about this revolution, and yet frequently their work is misrepresented in some ethical or pressure-group controversy, while publicity is given to medical media events of little genuine relevance to the health and welfare of women and their children.

This book puts things right. Wendy Cooper has the gift of communication in large measure and actually listens to the right doctors. The result is a reliable, factually correct account of the present state of medical knowledge as it applies to women. Everything is here, from cloning to pubic lice, and all presented with a maturity and balance born of genuine understanding.

Introduction:
A good time to be a woman

If ever there was a good time and a good place to be born a woman, it is here and now, in the Western world in the second half of the twentieth century.

Back in the sixties, Harold Macmillan coined the phrase, 'You've never had it so good.' Those words have come to have a slightly hollow ring in the present context of economic crisis, world inflation and unemployment. But there is one area in which they really do apply. The female of the species has never had it so good, not since *Homo sapiens* lumbered over the evolutionary horizon more than one million years ago.

For the first time ever, women are approaching something like equal opportunity with men. It is there for them to grasp in education, training, jobs, professions, promotion and pay, in principle, if not entirely in practice. With all this comes, or *should* come, improved confidence, improved status and associated economic, social and sexual freedom.

But these things will only prove possible and will only come about if women also avail themselves of the other fundamental freedom they are now being increasingly offered. This is biological freedom.

Biological freedom means exactly what it says – freedom from both the regular and the occasional tyranny which female biology by its very nature imposes. 'Biological Lib' is more important and more basic than any other form of liberation, because without it women are unable to exploit fully or enjoy the other freedoms for which they have fought.

But it should be said at once that Biological Liberation does not involve, as some of the extremist Women's Lib credo seems to do, any denial of womanhood or the feminine role. On the contrary, it embraces joyful recognition of what it means to be a woman, with all the pleasures, responsibilities and fulfilment inherent in our sexual and maternal natures. But it allows us to be in control of our natural female functions, instead of being at their mercy and dominated by them.

In my book *No Change: A Biological Revolution for Women* I concentrated on the way modern medicine can now help women during and after the menopause, *if* they wish it and *if* they need it, by replacing the oestrogen failing ovaries can no longer produce. Already this modern medical lifeline has brought biological liberation to thousands of older women.

In this book I want to look at the earlier part of a woman's life and the way medicine can help during the fertile years, from the time the ovaries establish the rhythmic ebb and flow of hormones that governs ovulation, to the time when they begin to falter and finally shut down, bringing an end to reproductive life.

To enable us to do this, we must understand as we go along something of our basic anatomy and of the hormonal tides that surge through us, influencing both our own lives and our ability to create new lives.

So many of a woman's problems and fears are linked to the very conditions which make her a woman. From her essential femininity comes the potential both for her greatest joy and fulfilment and also for her deepest fears and worries.

There are many women who are concerned, rightly and responsibly, with effective contraception and preventing unwanted children. Yet there are others (an amazing one in six) whose concern and sometimes deep agony is rooted in the apparent inability to achieve the longed-for family. In both cases we shall be looking at the choices now available, at new methods just around the corner, and most especially at the new hopes and positive successes involved in the latest exciting work on infertility.

There are so many medical lifelines now for women, so many advances in endocrinology, with accurate methods of assessing hormone levels, that new treatments are becoming available all the time for conditions which in the past women either had to tolerate or, at best, alleviate through pain-killers and tranquillizers.

More and more, modern medicine is tackling the root causes of women's complaints, and so we will also be looking at the latest ways of dealing with menstrual disorders – in particular pre-menstrual tension – and those other so-called 'female ailments' which are associated with the delicate and ever-changing balance of female hormones.

We will also be trying together to get a clear picture of most of the physical problems, big or small, that women worry about, from puberty onwards. So often simply understanding them can alleviate the fear. The modern woman really seems to want to know about her body, how it works and how sometimes modern drugs and techniques can help it to work better.

This avid and, I believe, healthy curiosity is already recognized and met to some extent by editors of newspapers and magazines, and by programme planners and producers in radio and television. Medical problems and medical progress now get tremendous coverage in all the media, much of it well done, but occasionally, because of limitations of space or time, the approach inevitably has to be superficial and the information over-simplified.

With a book there is a greater chance to go into detail, and the information is there for reference if and when you want it. The very length and permanence of a book allows research in depth and justifies talking to the leading doctors in specialist areas of medical knowledge. This I have done wherever possible, so that the views expressed are usually not mine, but those of experienced and responsible doctors. They are, however, 'translated', if that is the appropriate term, into our language – the language of ordinary people rather than physicians. Obviously the correct medical terms must be used, but these are usually explained in the text.

This book will be trying to get rid of some of the old wives' tales and damaging, unfounded folklore which can still linger on to mislead and sometimes frighten otherwise intelligent women. It does not say much for the level of school sex education that girls can still believe, as some do, that intercourse standing up cannot result in pregnancy; that you cannot get pregnant the first time; that *immediately* you are on the Pill you are safe; or that the so-called 'safe period' really is safe for most women.

Quite obviously this book (nor indeed any other book) could not or should not ever try to be a doctor-substitute. On the contrary, it should only try to help you to help your doctor so that, in turn, he or she can better help you. What you understand about *your* body should enable you to recognize more easily when anything is not quite right, and pinpoint symptoms which may be valuable to your doctor in correct diagnosis and treatment. It should also make possible a limited degree of self-help, so that you can supplement regular medical check-ups with your own more frequent and routine observations, particularly in such matters as breast examination.

So, between us, let's take the fear out of being female, the mystery out of medicine and the dread out of doctors. This book will strive to tell you what medicine can do for you now and what future developments promise. But it will also help, I hope, towards a better relationship between you and your doctor, increasing your confidence in your dealings with him, and increasing your pleasure in the very rewarding business of being a woman.

1 . You and your body

I feel slightly apologetic about starting this book with information which some readers will inevitably regard as too elementary. They will assume, as I once did, that through biology and sex education in our secondary schools every woman emerges with at least a working knowledge of her own anatomy, which is later augmented by the frank and open discussion we are all supposed to indulge in in our so-called permissive society, and by the flood of medical information in the media.

I can only say that from conversations with hundreds of women, from their letters and from the experiences of doctors, nurses and health visitors, it is clear that at least some women, far from becoming familiar with their own bodies, remain apprehensive strangers. They are on reasonably intimate terms, of course, with the outer surface and contours, taking good care of skin and hair and figure. But they are rather like some women drivers, who may keep their cars clean and polished, but still know nothing about what goes on under the bonnet.

At least that machine, the human body, comes in two varieties, which adds considerably to the spice of life. Despite some blurring of the sexual roles in recent years, there are anatomical, hormonal and functional differences between male and female. Men and women are not the same – they are not even equal, each having their strength and their weaknesses–but they are essentially complementary.

All the same, few would argue that of the two varieties of human machine, the female is the most marvellous and the most complex. Yet until quite recently, under the influence of patriarchal societies and religions (reinforced in the last century by Freud and his psychological theories), women have been held to be the weaker sex physically, intellectually and sexually. Twentieth-century medicine and, above all, the new understanding of hormones, together with modern statistics and records, have shown this assessment to be wrong in every respect.

Freud's view of women as an inferior form of mutilated male, castrated and doomed to envy superior male sexuality and covet the missing penis, has proved as wrong as the long-cherished belief that the male was the basic sex. We now know that the female is the prototype human form and that, left to itself, every foetus would turn toward the female. Only the powerful and continuous intervention of the male sex hormones, the androgens, effect the differentiation which results in a boy baby.

Producing a new human being (at least up to now) has required the usually pleasurable cooperation of male and female, whose marvellous but different machinery is designed for a satisfactory fit and a satisfactory outcome.

The fascinating process of conception will be traced in a later chapter, but for the moment, so that the rest of the book will be comprehensible, we need briefly and simply to go through the basic female anatomy and how it works. It should be quite painless. In fact you might even enjoy it, because you will find you are more intricate and wonderful than you ever suspected.

The female form

Our starting point is the fact that the human female is a mammal. That means that our young are born alive, as opposed to being hatched, and that our babies (at least in the natural state) are suckled at the breast.

At once this dictates certain physical characteristics. Although on average as adults we only achieve 85 per cent of the weight of the male, the pelvis (which is the bony cavity made up of the hips and lower bones of the spine) has to be relatively broader than a man's to allow a baby to pass from inside our body out into the world. All other measurements are usually smaller than those of a man, with the exception of the top of the thigh; our bones in general are smaller, lighter and less dense and our muscles, too, are smaller and less powerful.

The additional width of the pelvis gives the female broader hips than shoulders – hence the typical female contour. But at all ages most women also carry a greater proportion of fat, especially in the buttocks, breasts and abdominal wall. This not only confers on us the ability to stay warmer longer in cold water and cold weather (which must be counted at least a marginal asset), but also gives us the rounded curves which appear to be a major sexual asset.

Of course, I suspect men only find the ins and outs of the female figure delicious and exciting because they are associated with sexual maturity. We should probably be grateful that it is all reasonably aesthetic and that our potential for sexual response and reproduction is not signalled by our turning bright red or purple in selected areas, as happens with some lower primates.

The whole subject of the norms and forms of sexual attraction is a fascinating one, and although we must not let it divert us for too long, it does have relevance to any consideration of what goes to make a woman. There is strong evidence that we all respond to and learn to like what we get, but this can be modified by acquired cultural influences.

So, there is a basic and universal male response to female curves, but on top of that the Arabs, for instance, account a double-chin on the credit side in assessing beauty in a woman. Eskimos and Kaffirs go for obese women, though the Kaffirs rationalize it by pointing out that a fat woman stands a better chance of weathering famine than a lean one. Hottentots and Bushmen go in for enormous buttocks, clearly bred in by sexual selection.

The breasts

Our own contemporary society places enormous importance on the breasts, preferably large, firm and upstanding, and they often play a primary part in sexual arousal. They not only excite the male but his response to them excites the woman, with the nipples becoming erect during or even in anticipation of love-making. In other cultures, however, often where breasts are normally left uncovered, they seem to have much less sexual significance.

The ideal of breast beauty also varies in time and space. In the Middle Ages, in our own part of the world, small and round breasts were preferred, while large breasts were considered ugly. Pendulous, hanging breasts always seem to have been regarded as rather undesirable in our society, yet in some primitive tribes they are highly prized, and again tend to be bred in by sexual selection to the gratification of the adults and also of the babies: the idea is that the breast is long enough to be slung over the shoulder so that the child can be suckled while being carried on the back.

In the Western world, perhaps the decorative and erotic value of breasts has been somewhat over-played and the functional use for breast-feeding under-played. The latest understanding of the importance and value of breast-feeding to our babies is dealt with later in the book. Meanwhile, it is reassuring to know that actual breast size has no relationship to the ability to breast-feed, nor to sexual potential. Small breasts can produce as much milk as large and the owner of them as much passion.

Breasts should have assumed their adult form by the mid-teens, but if there is failure to develop medical treatment can now help. If there are associated menstrual problems, the chances are additional oestrogen is needed and will help the growth of the breast ducts. These milk ducts grow inwards from the nipple, dividing into smaller ducts and tiny milk-secreting areas called alveoli. If the problem is *not* hormonal, it is worth trying a better diet to encourage a better fat deposit, or possibly exercises to strengthen the pectoral muscle which supports the breast and thus helps to improve posture.

While oral oestrogen in the quantities a doctor may prescribe can often help, the small amounts contained in costly oestrogen creams will certainly not make your breasts grow – but is positively guaranteed to reduce your bank balance. For the adult woman who is really unable to come to terms with being flat-chested, plastic surgeons are sometimes prepared to insert silicone or other plastic moulds, but as cases of cancer have followed in a few instances, it is not something to be done without careful thought and good medical advice. Also, in the end it may be self-defeating. One young male who discussed his own reactions very frankly told me that when dating a young actress who had looked superb on the stage, he found later that what looked right certainly did not feel right. The presence of silicone breasts not only came to him as an awful shock but a total 'turn-off' and the evening was a disaster for both of them.

Fortunately nature itself can often provide an answer in the longer run through pregnancy, which leads to considerable growth of the ducts and the alveoli, particularly if the mother breast-feeds her baby.

Judging from the pictures of gorgeous girls which these days fill our popular newspapers, modern taste finds no breasts too big to be beautiful, but perhaps the really outsize types are less desirable and convenient as we get older and they become less firm. A well-designed, well-fitting bra is usually the answer, but sometimes in extreme cases surgery is performed to reduce them. For the woman with firm breasts there is certainly no need to wear a bra unless she feels more comfortable or more attractive in one. During the later stages of pregnancy, and afterwards if a woman is breast-feeding, it is advisable to wear a bra day and night, to avoid the increased weight of the breasts stretching the supporting tissues.

Nipples

The nipple contains muscle fibres which normally become erect on stimulation or exposure to cold. Occasionally a woman may have what is termed 'inverted' nipples, which do not respond in this way. This need be of no concern unless they still fail to evert during pregnancy and the expectant mother is planning to breast-feed.

In this case she should draw her doctor's attention to the problem so that treatment using a breast-pump or suction cup can be started. Once the nipple is drawn out, it should be rolled between the fingers; the process should be repeated regularly twice a day for some months if necessary. Nipple inversion suddenly acquired later in life should always be reported to your doctor, and more will be included about this in a later chapter, where we shall be dealing with routine self-examination of breasts.

Body hair

Hair under the arms and in the pubic and genital area is normal in a mature woman. Its growth is triggered by the sex hormones at puberty; long before anyone had heard of a hormone this association between body hair and sexual maturity was happily recognized. It led to the wide use of hair as a fertility symbol all over the ancient world and still to this day among some primitive cultures. By what psychoanalysts term 'displacement', the same sort of significance became attached to head hair, and long loose hair accordingly tended to symbolize sexuality and sexual licence, while cropped or concealed hair or a shaven head symbolized puritanism, discipline and even punishment.

Culture, conditioning and fashion again can affect attitudes to body hair as they can to body shape. In some races where body hair is naturally sparse it is considered ugly and any that does grow tends to be removed. The Japanese, the Dodingo tribe of Uganda, the Tobrian Islanders and many South American Indians all practise depilation as, long ago, did the Egyptians, the Greeks and the Romans, the fashion spreading from one culture to another. But from the Middle Ages, most Europeans have shown a fine appreciation of body hair, with writers as far apart in time and style as Shakespeare and D. H. Lawrence making the fact abundantly clear.

Even today, fashions regarding body hair vary not only from country to country but from woman to woman. While most of us choose to remove hair from our legs, in general French and Italian women prefer to leave underarm hair, while in Great Britain most women get rid of it. Few of us, however, seem to have taken up Mary Quant's advice to trim and shape our pubic hair to give a heart-shaped effect!

Excess hair

The one kind of body hair no woman welcomes is what we term excess hair, usually on the face. Where this is simply genetic in origin, little can be done about it except through electrolysis. But quite often the follicles, which we all possess, are triggered by a hormone imbalance, with a swing toward too much of the male hormone, testosterone. On rare occasions this can stem from a male-hormone-producing tumour of the ovary and the answer then has to be surgery. But almost always sudden onset of facial hair, indicating a change in the balance between oestrogen and the male hormones, androgens, which every woman produces in small amounts, can be either treated with oestrogen or an anti-androgen.

Hair around the nipple is another common condition which worries some women, but this has no significance and can be removed simply either by tweezers, razor or depilatory cream.

The genitals

The vulva

This is the name given to a woman's external genital organs, shown in Figure 1. The double set of lips or labia are designed

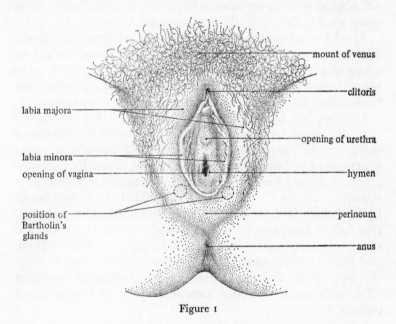

Figure 1

to protect the entrance to the vagina and uterus and other vital internal organs (Figure 2). In addition to the large lips (labia majora) and small lips (labia minora) which guard the body against invasion by undesirable foreign organisms, the vulva also includes the clitoris, the female equivalent of the male penis. Although much smaller, it is highly sensitive in its response to sexual stimulation and excitement and, like the penis, becomes filled with blood during arousal.

When not erect the clitoris is almost completely covered by a foreskin or prepuce. Between this and the labia minora are glands which produce a white fluid which tends to thicken and become soapy if it is not removed by careful washing. Because of its consistency it is actually called smegma, which is Greek for soap; in conjunction with the whole warm, moist environment, it can offer an ideal home for bacteria and yeasts which may cause itching, burning and inflammation, leading in turn to painful intercourse (dyspareunia). Careful washing of the vulva as part of normal hygiene can help to avoid these problems, but strong soaps, disinfectants and deodorant sprays are not a good idea. Some women have allergic reactions to them when used in this specially sensitive area.

Also lying between the labia minora are two pea-sized glands, known as Bartholin's glands, which supply some of the mucus acting as a lubricant in intercourse. There is also the small opening of the urethra, the outlet for urine. Below that and nearer the back outlet, or anus, is the larger entrance to the vagina.

In most, but by no means all, virgin girls this entrance is partially closed by a fold of membrane called the hymen or maidenhead. This varies in elasticity and has one or more apertures in it, but as the name implies it is usually stretched and torn during the first penetration for sexual intercourse. It should be mentioned that just a few girls have a very tough hymen which will not easily permit penetration. As a precaution before marriage or a first sexual experience, a medical check-up is often a good idea because it can reveal this condition and prevent a frustrating and wretched introduction to lovemaking, which can in some cases have a lasting and damaging effect on a woman's ability ever to respond or to experience orgasm.

The vagina and internal female organs (Figure 2)

The name vagina comes from the Latin word for sheath, but this hardly conveys the amazing nature of this muscular passage. Usually only about 4 in. (9 cm) long and 1 in. in diameter, the vagina is still capable of distension during sexual arousal to accommodate the largest male penis, and during childbirth to allow passage of the baby into the world.

It lies with the bladder in front of it and the rectum (back-

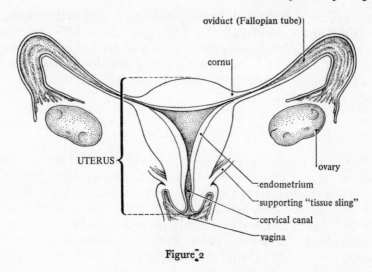

Figure 2

passage) behind it, sloping backward and upwards to join the cervix or neck of the womb. Not only is the healthy vagina so miraculously elastic, but it also has a built-in, self-cleansing mechanism. The walls of the vagina in a mature woman are some thirty cells thick and the outer layer of these are shed constantly, providing material which friendly, waiting bacilli then convert into lactic acid, which kills any contaminating germs.

In childhood the walls of the vagina are thin and this process does not take place, but fortunately at that time there is little risk of contamination to combat. After the menopause, unless a woman receives oestrogen-replacement therapy, the walls again become thin and the older woman can then have less protection against infection and inflammation. Hormone Replacement Therapy (HRT), now widely used to treat menopause and post-menopausal problems, restores the vagina to its pre-menopausal state, making it once again healthy and lubricating. This prevents the vaginal atrophy which can otherwise often occur. Fortunately, even when this has set in and has resulted in painful intercourse, HRT can rapidly reverse the changes; so it is never too late to consult a doctor if there are problems with vaginal dryness.

Oestrogen is the chief female sex hormone and matures the

cells of the vaginal wall. Examination of the cells of the vagina, stained and viewed under a microscope, can actually indicate the oestrogen level at any given time. The doctor calculates the ratio of mature cells to immature cells revealed by the smear test and slide, giving the patient's oestrogen level; this is called the Maturation Index.

The cervix

The word cervix simply means neck, and describes the narrow cavity or neck of the womb which reaches down into the vagina. Because it is so easily accessible for examination it is particularly important in the detection of any early changes in cells which might lead to cancer if untreated; this is discussed in detail later in the book. The narrow channel which widens into the uterus or womb is called the cervical canal.

The uterus

Popularly called the womb, the uterus is even more remarkable than the vagina. Before pregnancy it is less than 4 in. (9 cm) in length and pear-shaped, measuring only 2½ in. (6 cm) at its widest point. Yet it can expand to enclose and protect a baby which may reach 20 in. (50 cm) in length.

Three strong muscular layers woven together form this tough but elastic container, and normally the uterus lies bent forward at an angle of ninety degrees to the vagina, resting on the bladder. As the bladder fills the uterus is pushed back and as the bladder empties it falls forward again. In just a few women (about 15 per cent) the uterus lies bent backward; this is called 'retroversion'. Once this was considered serious and sometimes corrected by surgery, but these days a 'tipped' uterus is recognized as unimportant and normal to many women. If it is considered that it may be a minor cause of infertility, then the patient may be advised to lie on her abdomen with her hips supported by a pillow for half an hour after intercourse in order to line up the sperm with the opening to the cervix. Intercourse in a rear-entry position may also be advised. Surgery is rarely used today unless there is associated endometriosis or pelvic inflammation, conditions which will be discussed later.

The endometrium

This is the name given to the inner lining of the womb. In contrast to the tough exterior, this is soft and rich in blood vessels and mucous glands, forming a nice, warm, moist nest for any baby which may be conceived.

The fallopian tubes

The body of the uterus, which is the name given to the broad upper part, narrows away on each side to join the fallopian tubes, also called oviducts, which gives a better clue to their purpose. As Figure 2 shows, these tubes lie in contact with the ovary on each side and the long finger-like processes catch the egg (or ovum) when it is expelled each month from the ovary, sweeping it on down hopefully to meet a male sperm, when conception may take place.

The ovaries

The two ovaries are really the female powerhouses. Almond-shaped and whitish in colour, they are only about 2 in. (4½ cm) long and less than an inch (2½ cm) thick. But even before a girl baby is born her ovaries already contain some 200000 egg cells from which yet another generation may come. The ovaries, however, are not only the long-term storehouse for the eggs, but also a fascinating and complex hormone factory, producing the female sex hormones which control the reproductive cycle and the rhythm of a woman's life.

2. The hormonal tides and menstruation

We have mentioned that the ovaries are factories for producing female hormones and have referred several times already to hormones and Hormone Replacement Therapy. So now we will try to describe what a hormone is and what it does. By definition a hormone is a substance secreted and released by glands into the blood stream to stimulate other glands, organs, and tissues into activity.

It is extraordinary how definitions almost invariably manage to make anything sound dull, and that one certainly fails to convey anything of the powerful and exciting nature of hormones, or the amazing and intricate tasks they perform.

The master gland is the pituitary, situated in the base of the skull, and it is sometimes likened to a conductor in the way it controls and orchestrates all the other glands. Apart from releasing a growth hormone which causes the spurt of growth at puberty, the pituitary is also responsible in the sexually mature woman for starting up the dazzling chain of events and an increased resultant hormonal ebb and flow which will form the pattern of her life during the fertile years.

Under the influence of the hypothalamus, a special part of the brain, the pituitary begins by secreting minute quantities of a hormone known as FSH, for follicle stimulating hormone – and that is exactly what it does. Less than one-millionth of an ounce a day of this powerful FSH is sufficient to awaken the dormant female egg cells, which have been lying quiescent and undisturbed inside the ovaries since before birth.

But now under the stimulus of FSH a fluid-filled follicle, rather like a tiny protective sac, forms round several of the awakened egg cells. Usually only one of these follicles actually goes on to grow and expand sufficiently to force its way through the surface of the ovary to appear as a sort of bubble. If, as happens on very rare occasions, *two* follicles succeed in doing this then the possibility exists for the conception of non-identical twins, assuming both of the two separate eggs are fertilized.

But first the growing follicles secrete more oestrogen to add to what the ovaries are already producing, and this rise in oestrogen signals to the uterus to start preparing a thick and welcoming lining, where any fertilized egg can become safely embedded and nourished.

By a form of feed-back mechanism, these rising levels of oestrogen are sensed by the pituitary, which responds by sending a second hormone called LH, or luteinizing hormone, whose strange name is explained later. When LH joins FSH around mid-cycle, their combined effect causes the follicle bubble on the outside of the ovary to burst, releasing the egg. When it does so, it makes quite a tear in the membrane covering the ovary; some women can actually feel this happen and experience a short, sharp pain. There is also a slight rise in temperature when ovulation occurs, and this can be detected by women and used both in trying to achieve conception or in trying to avoid it, as obviously it heralds the time when there is the best chance of sperm and egg coming together.

After the egg is released, the fronds or fingers at the end of the fallopian tube gently catch the egg and waft it slowly into the fallopian cavity where fertilization may or may not occur.

Either way, the now empty follicle collapses and the LH acts on the cell walls to turn them yellow, forming the *corpus luteum*, or yellow body, from the latin word *luteus*, meaning yellow – hence the name, luteinizing hormone. This change of colour also signifies a change in the cell activity because the *corpus luteum* now produces not only oestrogen but also the other important female hormone, progesterone. Again the name indicates the function, for it means pro-gestation or pro-pregnancy; progesterone is known as the pregnancy hormone. Its main job is to preserve and modify the uterine lining, inducing it to secrete a nutritious fluid to nourish any fertilized egg during the time it takes to become implanted in the lining of the womb.

If conception does *not* take place, after about twelve to fourteen days the *corpus luteum* dies and the supply of progesterone is shut off, while the level of oestrogen also drops. These changes inform the waiting womb that no baby has been conceived this time, and so the lining that has been built up is allowed to flow away taking with it the unfertilized egg. This is what we call menstruation.

Myths about menstruation

Now that we understand what menstruation is and why it happens, it should be far easier to accept it as a natural and unembarrassing event, certainly nothing of which women need to feel shy or ashamed.

Any lingering feelings of that sort almost certainly stem from old myths and superstititions common to many cultures, where menstruating women were regarded as contaminating and even dangerous. These beliefs were rooted in ignorance and fear, stemming partly from the association of blood with injuries and death, and partly from the idea that the monthly loss of blood was a form of purging in which a woman got rid of unclean substances.

It is amazing how long such old superstititons can survive. As comparatively recently as 1878, the *British Medical Journal* carried two reports of hams being spoiled because they had been cured by menstruating women.

Another old idea which took a long time to die was that menstruation was somehow triggered by the moon. This was due to the coincidence of the twenty-eight-day cycle; as recently as 1938, American medical students could still read in an authoritative textbook on obstetrics: 'over 71 per cent of women menstruate every twenty-eight days and the majority during the new moon'. The absurdity of all women menstruating at the same time seems to have struck no one. It's certainly not true when they are separated and dispersed, but there is considerable and growing evidence that women living together in all-women communities, such as colleges or women's prisons, gradually adjust their cycles to exhibit a sort of communal periodicity. It's a strange finding and hard to account for in medical terms. But it can also happen within some small family units. One doctor told me that after his young daughter began to menstruate regularly, her cycles began to exactly match those of her mother. This continued all the time she was living at home, but when she went away to boarding school, her cycles gradually shifted over two years to match the dormitory pattern. Now the family has moved and the daughter is able to attend day-school and live at home, once again her menstrual periods have adjusted to match those of her mother.

Most of us are familiar with that old euphemism for menstruation, 'the curse', and it is something which mothers would be wise to avoid; it is far better and healthier for girls to be taught to welcome menstruation as a sign of growing up and entering into womanhood – something of which to be proud rather than to dread. And while we are about it we can dismiss those other old wives' tales such as the notion that washing hair during a period leads to increased loss or colds or even to pneumonia. There is absolutely no truth in such ideas, so that unless the menstrual loss is really exceptionally heavy, girls today quite rightly refuse to let this natural and regular occurrence affect their activities, and walk, run, ride and even swim, doing just exactly what they feel like doing. Apart from the fact that it is a little more messy, there is also nothing harmful about having intercourse during menstruation if both partners find it acceptable. For some women it can even be a time of heightened desire.

Having argued for this sensible approach, it still has to be said that there are some women who are unable to take it all so easily in their stride. Painful menstruation and what is termed pre-menstrual tension will be considered later.

Protection

I made the point at the beginning of this book that women today are lucky and this certainly applies to protection during the period of menstrual flow. It's not really so very long ago that women had to use bits of cloth – bulky, uncomfortable and held precariously in position with bits of tape round the waist. One English name for menstruation was 'the rags', and no wonder. The wretched bits of cloth had to be washed and boiled and re-used, and with a large family of girls and no washing machines it must have been a wretched and time-consuming business.

In contrast, today it is all made so easy for us. There are sanitary pads of easily disposable materials, and the latest types adhere without tapes or belts. Better still in many ways is the internal tampon, as this eliminates the chafing that an external pad can sometimes cause. There is absolutely no truth in the idea that it is dangerous to collect menstrual blood in the vagina or that tampons can cause infection. They can, of course, if they are left in and forgotten; most gynaecologists are familiar with the frantic consultation from a woman with a strange discharge, who on examination proves to be harbouring an old tampon.

Even young girls just starting periods can usually use the smallest junior-sized tampon. When first learning to insert these a liberal coating of vaseline or similar lubricant is helpful. For the woman who has a few days of heavy loss, a tampon *and* a pad may be necessary.

Recently attempts were made in America to introduce a 'deodorant tampon', but as with spray deodorants there is a chance that these may kill off useful protective bacteria so that harmful ones are thereby allowed to flourish.

What is normal?

The amount of loss during a menstrual period can vary tremendously not just from woman to woman but for the same woman at different times, so it is difficult to lay down guidelines. Periods first begin any time between the ages of ten and sixteen (with average age of onset being thirteen). Statistics indicate that 95 per cent of girls start their periods when they reach a body weight of between forty-five and forty-nine kilos (around seven stone).

There is often very scanty bleeding and considerable irregularity; but in those early years this is of no significance. If menstrual periods have not started by the sixteenth birthday, it is a good idea to consult a doctor. Usually the answer is found in a prescription for female hormones to prod the lazy ovaries into action.

One of the results of delayed maturity in both sexes can be over-tall girls or boys. Obviously, few boys worry about being extra tall, but to a girl this can be an embarrassment. Puberty causes the growing bones to fuse and so further growth tends to be prevented. Because of this, deliberately *inducing* the onset of puberty can be very important where there is real fear of a girl growing abnormally tall.

As in all good medicine there has to be proper assessment of risk and benefit. Preventing a girl from growing too tall can be important, but there can also be problems of psychological damage for some girls having to cope with over-early puberty.

Occasionally what is termed 'precocious puberty' *can* occur naturally and this is more common in girls than in boys. In very rare instances there can be an obvious physical cause, such as a tumour which, if found, must be dealt with before other treatment is used; but often there is no obvious reason for the maturing mechanism starting to function too soon, and so treatment consists of damping down the pituitary with another hormone, a synthetic version of progesterone called Provera.

This use of hormones to help control abnormal growth or lack of growth in the young is another very new lifeline;[1] it should be emphasized that it is a rare problem, but one which parents are beginning to realize can benefit from medical help. Abnormal tallness – or the opposite of stunted growth – should not be confused with just being a bit taller than average or being what is called 'small normal'. As an example, about three children in every one hundred may be 'small normal', but only one child in every thousand falls into the abnormal category which requires medical help.

The earlier such help is sought the better, particularly in the case of possible stunted growth. Dr Paul Rayner, consultant paediatrician at Birmingham's famous Children's Hospital, showed me the growth charts for 'Mary', who at the age of five measured only 79 cm (31 in.) in height, comparable to an eighteen-month-old baby. In her case the reason was found to be the most common one in this country – thyroid deficiency, which can be easily diagnosed and treated with thyroid extract. Now, at the age of thirteen, Mary has caught up with her normal height.

In the underdeveloped world, of course, the most common reason for lack of proper growth is poor nutrition but, as Dr Rayner explained, that is not the case here: 'Apart from thyroid deficiency the next most common reason in this country for stunted growth is deficiency of actual growth hormone.'

This condition again is very rare and affects only one in every ten thousand children. Dr Rayner has told me that human growth hormone cannot be synthesized, so 'we are striving to organize a donor system with donor cards, as is already done with kidneys and corneas'.

As more parents become aware that abnormally stunted growth can be treated, they are coming forward for medical help, so that obviously more human pituitary growth hormone material is going to be needed if the necessary help is to be given.

Although it is important to seek help early, Dr Rayner also made the point that chronological age is not the real determining factor. 'It's the relationship between bone age and the actual age and the growth potential in reserve which is important,' he explained. 'A boy or girl of even twenty might still be able to be treated, if the bone age on investigation proved to be that of a ten- or twelve-year-old.'

I am sure it is important that parents should know about these problems, however rare they are, but fortunately for most of us puberty comes at the right time and growth follows a normal pattern.

In most women a regular menstrual pattern finally emerges of around twenty-eight days with the first day of loss counting as day one. But in some women periods are more frequent, coming as often as every twenty-one days, while in others they can be as far apart as thirty-five days. Anything in this range is considered normal, but if bleeding lasts more than seven days or is excessive or painful, your doctor should be consulted. Hormonal treatment for a few months will often put things right or, sometimes, if a routine gynaecological examination does not provide the answer, a thyroid test may be advised to determine whether supplemental thyroid or iodine medication may be required to regulate the periods.

The woman who wants or needs to change the date of an expected menstrual period to fit with holiday or honeymoon nowadays can be helped quite simply to do so by her doctor. With use of either the contraceptive pill or of oestrogen in one form or another, the cycle can be adjusted. The only difficulty arises once ovulation has occurred in mid-cycle. After that it is difficult to bring the period on earlier, but it can still be delayed by as much as a week. In view of this it is obviously wise to give your doctor one or two months' warning when a single special date is looming up, to enable him to adjust your cycle with no problem.

Delayed menstruation

There is a saying, 'Time and tide wait for no man,' illustrating the inexorable nature of ocean tides and passing time. But hormonal tides in women are not quite so reliable or predictable and far more often it is we who anxiously await for both time and tide to reassure us we are not pregnant.

If periods have always been regular, then a missed period most likely does indicate conception, particularly if birth control has not been used. But this is not always the case, as illness, anxiety, fatigue, emotional disturbance, excitement or even sometimes just climatic change can temporarily cause a hormone imbalance and upset the natural rhythm.

It is not really too surprising if you remember that the whole process after all starts in that part of the brain called the hypothalamus, which in turn controls the pituitary master gland. There can clearly be a two-way process at work, with hormonal levels influencing emotions and emotions also affecting hormone production via a feed-back system.

Usually when a period is delayed and a check-up shows no pregnancy, there has been a failure to ovulate. This means there has been no developing follicle to add its own quota of oestrogen, and the amount coming from the ovaries alone has not been enough to trigger menstruation at the right time. Finally, however, the inevitable and gradual build-up of the lining of the womb under oestrogen stimulation does reach the stage when it has become so thick it just has to start shedding, and then bleeding eventually starts.

Fortunately for women these days there is no need for long anxious waiting and worrying over possible pregnancy. Not only is birth control available, efficient and free, which should eliminate anxiety in the normal way, but if for any reason pregnancy is suspected it can be checked quickly, easily and early. This is explained in detail in later chapters.

It is sometimes helpful to know the terms doctors use even if we do not use them ourselves, and failure to menstruate is called *amenorrhoea*. Primary amenorrhoea is absence of menstruation in a growing girl, and if periods have not started by the age of sixteen, as already indicated a doctor should be consulted. Usually the sluggish ovaries are prodded into action quite simply with hormonal treatment and only very rarely is there a more fundamental problem.

Secondary amenorrhoea is when menstruation has been successfully established and then for some reason stops. As we have seen there can be many reasons for this quite apart from pregnancy. Sometimes the emotional upset of going away from home to university or to a new job can be enough to affect hormonal output temporarily. In fact 25 per cent of girls first entering university are reported to miss up to three periods just as a result of excitement and change of environment.

During the Second World War the term 'Kriegs amenorrhoea', or war amenorrhoea, was coined for the complete lapse of periods which occurred in many women during their time in the fearful concentration camps. No doubt the terrible conditions and stress were responsible because menstruation often ceased before the starvation diet could have had time to take effect.

Women and girls may often miss their periods after having been raped, which obviously adds to their outrage and upset the fear of pregnancy. Needless to say a doctor should always be consulted in such cases, however humiliating it may be for a woman to talk about what has happened.

Anorexia nervosa is another very common cause for secondary amenorrhoea. In fact, a very interesting survey carried out recently at St Mary's Hospital Medical School, London, found that out of 170 consecutive patients with amenorrhoea, thirty-nine had it directly as a result of weight loss; of these, twenty-four cases were *firmly* diagnosed as caused by anorexia nervosa, with many of the others as possibles.[2]

It is a disorder which mainly affects adolescent girls and has perhaps been best described as 'wilful pursuit of thinness through self-starvation'. It may not sound too serious but it can actually lead to death and does so in a quite alarming proportion of cases. In one follow-up study quoted in *Woman's Body* (Paddington Press), four out of the thirty women died.

Anorexia nervosa usually starts innocently enough with dieting, either because the girl really is overweight or simply believes that she is. It then develops insidiously into a morbid fear of fatness and leads to extreme and ugly emaciation, strangely enough rarely recognized by the girl herself. The weight loss is not only accompanied by loss of menstruation but by constipation and discoloration of the skin.

The reasons are highly complex and not fully understood, though it is believed that anorexia nervosa cases fall into two types. In one case the woman seems to want to negate her own sexuality – to be afraid of it – and in the other, genuinely to believe that slimming will make her more attractive. Sexual problems are usually involved, often together with quite unwarranted lack of self-confidence or self-esteem. Again sometimes it can involve part of the whole adolescent drive toward independence or a rejection of family and parental norms, while sometimes thinness itself simply seems to be the desired goal. Whatever the reason, the condition needs recognition and treatment, both on the psychiatric and medical level. This is not always as easy as it would appear, because girls suffering from anorexia disorder will go to extraordinary lengths to hide the fact that they are not eating. One very good-looking girl of sixteen, whom I knew personally, came to resemble a survivor from Belsen over a period of some months, during which time her bewildered family was fooled into believing she was having good school dinners. Not only was she never eating at school, but even at home she was managing to secrete a lot of the food put in front of her, smuggling it away in handkerchiefs and pockets.

Severe cases invariably require a stay in hospital with drug therapy and encouragement toward a high-calorie diet. Bed rest is part of the treatment and the patient is allowed up only after reaching near-normal weight, which can take between one and three months.

Dysmenorrhoea means painful and difficult menstruation. This does not usually start to occur until a few years after periods begin and then usually only when ovulation has taken place. But some 50 per cent of women complain of dysmenorrhoea at some stage of their life, with the peak years between seventeen and twenty-five. This is probably because the cervical canal is narrower than it will be later in life and the uterus has to contract more forcibly to expel menstrual blood.

If these so-called menstrual cramps are so severe that they are not relieved by mild pain-killers, then a doctor should be consulted.

The oral contraceptive is often prescribed by doctors to prevent or treat dysmenorrhoea, but for a young girl still at school, parents (or sometimes grandparents) find it difficult to accept treatment which they feel may encourage sexual freedom. In such cases, fortunately, today other hormone treatment, which does *not* inhibit ovulation, is available.

Endometriosis

In very rare cases menstrual blood may flow back into the pelvic cavity; if this goes on over a period of years there is a chance of *endometriosis* developing. This is a condition where cells of the endometrium (lining of the womb) are deposited and become grafted to other organs. Although not in their right place, they still respond to hormone influence and start bleeding during the menstrual period. The presence of the cells and the unwanted bleeding in the wrong areas can set up irritation and pain. It can also cause infertility or even sterility.

Where endometriosis does occur it can fortunately be treated with continuous hormone treatment. Occasionally, a dilation and curettage (D and C) has been used to widen the cervical opening to allow easier menstrual flow, on the assumption that pressure in the uterus has forced the blood backwards into the body cavity. A pregnancy, of course, has the same effect, so that young mothers are least likely to suffer from painful menstruation or the risk of endometriosis.

Pelvic congestion

This is another condition some women complain about because of feelings of pressure in the pelvis, backache and a general feeling of being uncomfortable and unwell. The symptoms are believed to be due to congestion of the pelvic organs with blood and sufferers do often have heavier periods. This condition can be associated also with feelings of sexual inadequacy and some doctors believe emotional stress can be involved. Obviously, if so, resolving the emotional problems or just talking about them can help but again hormone treatment can also provide relief.

Perhaps the golden rule with menstruation is to become familiar with your own special individual pattern of loss and timing. Because all of us are individuals with individual chemistry and hormone levels, there is little point in worrying about comparisons with other women. What is a heavy period for one woman is a normal one for another. The sensible rule is to consult your doctor only if there is real pain associated with your period or if you note a sudden change in the usual bleeding pattern.

Obviously, toward the end of fertile life this is going to happen with us all, and indeed some women begin to encounter symptoms of the change of life, including flushes, even before menstruation is affected. Usually the ovaries begin to falter in the late forties with final menstruation coming around the age of fifty or fifty-one. But in some women it can come much earlier, even in the mid-thirties; often the age at which your mother ceased to menstruate can give you a clue about when it will happen to you, as there is an underlying genetic control at work.

At whatever age the menopause comes today there is nothing to worry about. For some women there are no problems anyway, but for others who suffer from severe flushes, sweats, depression or vaginal atrophy (dryness and shrinkage), modern medicine has an effective answer in Hormone Replacement Therapy, commonly known as HRT.[3] This involves replacing the oestrogen which failing ovaries can no longer produce and it rapidly eliminates menopause miseries. Prescription data in 1977 showed over 200000 women already on this treatment in the UK.[4] But the whole concept is fully explained in my book, *No Change*, which looks specifically at this later period of a woman's life. Right now we are concerned with the fertile years and the pleasures and the problems these can bring.

3. Pre-menstrual syndrome: new understanding and new treatment

Throughout history women have earned themselves a reputation for being at times emotional, weepy and unpredictable. 'Fickle, fair and hard to please' has been the male verdict. Few men have understood the violent mood swings and personality changes women undergo. Only recently has medicine begun to recognize the importance of hormone levels and hormone imbalance not just to the body but to the mind.

Some women are so affected by hormone imbalance that they go through a period in the second half of each cycle when they suffer from what has been called 'pre-menstrual tension' severely enough to make life hell even for considerate partners and families. A librarian writes:

Each month after ovulation I begin 12–15 days of increasing misery. My breasts and abdomen start to swell and I search out what I call my 'fat' clothes. I have one extraordinary day when I'm totally devoid of any kind of feeling except almost ungovernable anger. The last time I threw a large *Oxford Dictionary* at my husband and wasn't a bit put out when the book split and fell to pieces, which is out of character as I both work with books and collect them as a hobby.

Maybe she collects husbands too, for the letter entirely fails to mention if she found her target or what happened to the poor man. It goes on:

The last few days of each cycle are mainly a tale of increasing incompetence: I fall over things; trip down stairs; drop books all over my library; ruin my cooking; talk strange gibberish and have an alarming tendency to cry copiously for no apparent reason. However, the very worst thing is the awful tenderness of my breasts, which is sometimes so bad I just sit down and cry about that too. It gets better the day before I start my period and clears up after about another three days. Suggestions when I have sought treatment in the past have been either ineffective or inappropriate – 'take more exercise', when I already belong to a gymnastics club, swimming club and a hockey team. Or, 'You'll be all right when you have a baby', when I was only a girl of 17. Now when I'm married and trying to conceive a child I am told 'You should go on the Pill'. I managed to get through university but dreaded exams falling before my period rather than after it. I do apologise for the resounding peals of self-pity but would be grateful for any help.

That letter encapsulates many of the problems which form the classic pattern of the pre-menstrual syndrome (PMS): the regularity of onset, the mixture of physical and psychological symptoms, the effect on the family, the adverse effect on examination results and the frustrations encountered in getting effective treatment.

Most women have a minor reaction to the fall in hormones which precedes menstruation. They may feel a little more tired, irritable and depressed, sometimes with an accompanying touch of backache, but it is something they can cope with because it usually only lasts for one or two days and then disappears with the start of a period.

At least this rather common mild version of PMS enables us to understand what it must be like for the less fortunate women whose experience is more severe and prolonged; coming every cycle with tyrannical regularity, often starting as much as ten or fourteen days before menstruation and persisting until it is well under way. The effect can be so intense that life is disrupted both at home and at work, and along with the woman herself the husband and family can come to dread the monthly misery involved.

The physical symptoms vary but usually include backache, sore breasts, headaches, abnormal lethargy and, often, a bloated feeling and weight gain caused by water retention. Sometimes there can be nausea and even vomiting.

While the physical symptoms vary from woman to woman and even from cycle to cycle in the same woman, the mental symptoms – mounting tension, irritability and black depression – are far more consistent. At such times women can, as the letter showed, become clumsy, emotional and accident-prone, giving way to bursts of illogical anger often vented on the family.

The effect of PMS on a normally equable wife can be so devastating that it is often the husband who forces her to see a doctor and who helps her and her GP to recognize the true cyclic nature of the problem. One husband described to me what he called the 'regular horrible personality change', and another referred to his much-loved wife as 'a sort of female Jekyll and Hyde'. Yet another, who was also a doctor, said, 'The only place for a woman at those times is down the garden.'

But the effects of PMS do not stop at the patient and her family. They affect society too and not just in terms of unhappy or broken marriages, children in care, absenteeism or reduced efficiency at work. It has been shown that more than 50 per cent of female crime, from shoplifting to baby-battering, takes place during the PMS phase.

In fact PMS was first recognized by criminologists rather than by doctors. Well over one hundred years ago a French survey on shoplifting (which we tend to think of as just a modern form of crime) showed that 63 per cent of the women offenders committed this sort of theft during their PMS phase. It was so completely accepted as a contributive factor in crime that under the French criminal code a woman who was clever enough to murder her husband during her PMS phase would get off, while another woman committing the same crime at a less judicious time would get the guillotine.

The association of PMS with female crime is now well substantiated in this country, too, and in modern records this shows very clearly, as does the fact that more than half the female suicides and admissions to mental and other hospitals also occur during the PMS part of the cycle. It is also the time when women are most subject to viral and bacterial infection and to recurrence of allergic conditions such as asthma.[5]

Any woman who has reason to suspect that she suffers from PMS should start by keeping a menstrual chart over two or three cycles and, if the symptoms prove to occur at the same time each month, she can then take this convincing evidence to her own doctor to help him in his own diagnosis.

It is the wide diversity of the symptoms which made the condition difficult to diagnose, and which has often led to symptomatic treatment only. Unless the woman herself, or sometimes someone close to her, recognizes the cyclic recurrence of the syndrome, it is hard for a doctor, possibly consulted irregularly only when things get really bad, to tie in the odd headaches, backache or depression with PMS. Water retention should certainly offer the strongest clue; strangely enough, while dismissing PMS as being all in the mind (as the menopause was once dismissed) doctors are forced to concede some physical aspect when they prescribe diuretics to combat water retention. But if they do not even realize the problem is a cyclic one, the chances are they will just prescribe pain-killers for headaches and anti-depressants or tranquillizers for the depression.

Many women feel very strongly about the way in which they are treated as neurotic if they dare to complain about PMS. Some 40 per cent of women consult their doctors at some time or other, but because the other 60 per cent of women do not suffer from PMS (or at least do not complain) too many doctors in the past have treated the ones who do as 'female nuisances'.

One 36-year-old woman wrote:

The headaches I experience at exactly the same time each month are so bad that for at least 48 hours I dare not even drive my car. The pain-killers I am prescribed just make me a dopey bad-tempered mother. It seems to me that PMS is treated as a 'neurotic female complaint' and you are made to feel guilty for wasting your GP's valuable time with something which he does not consider a physical illness. He simply tells me it will probably stop after the menopause, but surely this is a long time for the family to suffer.

Another woman made the point that severe PMS symptoms in themselves are enough to make a woman become neurotic. She wrote: 'Who wouldn't be neurotic after five years in which there has only been one week in each month when I have felt human or normal?'

As with the menopause, it is not entirely easy to separate built-in neurotic tendencies from mental symptoms triggered by hormone imbalance – each can tend to aggravate the other. But an interesting new study recently carried out by Dr A. W. Clare of the Institute of Psychiatry in London found that although 75 per cent of a general practice sample of 521 women complained of at least one pre-menstrual symptom, at least half of them were psychologically completely healthy. On the other hand he found that most women who complained of psychological difficulties also complained of PMS. He is now carrying out further work to explore the relationship between psychiatric, social and hormonal variables.

Although in the past PMS has been largely treated symptomatically, as the menopause once was, the actual clues implicating a hormonal basis are big enough to fall over.

There is the fact that PMS starts for the first time either at or after puberty, or following childbirth – both periods when the hormone balance is disturbed. There is the seemingly miraculous disappearance of PMS with onset of menstruation or pregnancy – both times when hormone levels are changing. There is the regularity with which true PMS strikes at the same time in the cycle – always in the second half when ovulation has occurred and brought the second female hormone, progesterone, into play. There is the fact that a drop in progesterone levels is already implicated in some forms of depression and tiredness and, yet again, the fact that many women feel better and suffer less from PMS when taking the combined progestogen and oestrogen pill.

Progestogen is the name given to any synthetic version of progesterone. The problem with pure progesterone is that it is destroyed in the digestive tract and it is, therefore, not practical to give it by mouth.

One British doctor, Katharina Dalton, has argued for years that PMS was rooted in a relative imbalance between progesterone and oestrogen levels and has claimed a success rate of between 80 and 90 per cent with pure progesterone treatment. Initially this had to be in the form of injections, which are both expensive and somewhat painful, but more recently it has become available as pessaries or suppositories.[6] Despite this easier method of administration, and despite a long, sustained and lonely battle over the years to get PMS recognized, diagnosed and correctly treated, few women have ever been offered pure progesterone or been told about the treatment by their doctors. Dr Dalton has told me that:

GPs actually try to argue that women will not accept pessaries and suppositories, that they don't like using them, but I can only say they have accepted them willingly enough for other medical purposes such as treating thrush and other local infections.

And I can only say that the women I have met and talked to, all sufferers from severe PMS, were desperate enough to have tried anything their doctors prescribed. Indeed they were desperate enough to respond to a small notice in *Good House-keeping* magazine, describing special trials of a new oral hormone treatment to take place at St Thomas's Hospital, London, and to travel sometimes hundreds of miles to take part.

For those first uncontrolled trials, suitable volunteers were selected from over 300 women who applied and came for an interview. On the assumption that neither injections, implants, pessaries nor suppositories are convenient to all women, the St Thomas's team, under Professor R. Taylor of the Obstetrics and Gynaecology Department, had been seeking a progestogen which could be taken by mouth and still prove effective in treating PMS. One synthetic progestogen called norethisterone gave good relief of breast discomfort but did not relieve fully the other symptoms, and finally Professor Taylor opted for one called dydrogesterone, chosen because of its close chemical and structural resemblance to pure progesterone. Given from the twelfth day to the twenty-fifth day (10 mg twice a day), a 72 per cent success rate was achieved in the preliminary trials.[7] (Ironically the only symptom which generally failed to respond was the breast discomfort which had been so well relieved by the different type of progestogen.) Single blind controlled trials with dydrogesterone and placebo are now under way, and meanwhile more and more GPs are starting to use this method of treatment, with considerable success reported.

But although dydrogesterone proved the most effective method, the St Thomas's team also had good results in cases where hormone assays showed no low level of progesterone. For these patients a simple vitamin B6 (pyridoxine) was used in divided doses from 40 mg daily up to, in a few cases, 100 mg daily. The treatment was begun three days before expected onset of PMS and also continued up to menstruation. Over half of the seventy patients treated in this way were found to benefit markedly, particularly in relief of headache, oedema (water retention) and bloatedness, but also of depression and irritability. The relief of headaches was especially striking, with 62 per cent completely relieved, 19 per cent markedly improved and 6 per cent improved. Pyridoxine has also been found to be beneficial in relieving depression associated with the Pill, and this is discussed in the chapter on contraception.[8]

The underlying causes of PMS are obviously more complex than the relatively straightforward oestrogen deficiency, known to underlie menopausal symptoms and to respond so clearly to oestrogen replacement.

Professor P. H. F. Giles out in Australia has already had good results with the use of pyridoxine, which seems to work by relieving the vitamin B deficiency associated with a disturbance of tryptophane metabolism. This is an amino acid which in turn can affect production of something called 5-hydroxy-tryptamine, a substance which acts as a chemical transmitter in the brain.[9]

It all sounds immensely complicated and it is, but the long names do not matter. What does matter is that it is known that lowered levels of this essential brain substance can cause depression. So it is not difficult to see how the chain reaction can start from a simple vitamin deficiency and, equally, how it can be prevented.

In other cases where progesterone levels are found to be low, the more common progesterone–oestrogen balance has to be put right. But there is yet a third possibility in PMS which involves another hormone called prolactin, the milk-producing hormone. In just a few women, raised levels of prolactin may be implicated and work is going on to treat these with a new drug called bromocriptine.[10]

So it is a complicated picture, but a new surge of interest and research is already producing practical results – one of the treatments usually works for individual PMS sufferers. All are designed to treat the root cause rather than just symptoms. Some doctors also achieve considerable success by prescribing the combined pill, which substitutes its own artificial hormone levels for the natural and obviously faulty levels in some PMS patients. But not all women with PMS want to be in a contra-ceptive state and in just a few women the combined pill can itself induce a form of depression as bad as the PMS it sets out to cure. This will be considered in more detail in Chapter 5.

One encouraging thing for women suffering from PMS is that at least there should not be the same resistance to hormonal treatment as menopause sufferers once encountered. Progesterone and progestogens appear to be well tolerated with few side-effects, and there are no lingering cancer fears to combat as in the case of oestrogens. But, more important, the fact that 60 per cent of women do *not* suffer from PMS should at least put it firmly in the realm of pathology. With the menopause happening sooner or later to *all* women, it was easy for some doctors to argue that it was 'natural' and something women must 'put up with'. It took a long time to convince these physicians that severe menopause symptoms could be so bad and so damaging that they could hardly be written off as physiological, but needed treating like any other symptoms, preferably by tackling the root cause.

Doctors can hardly argue that PMS is natural, yet believe it or not two recently tried to do so. Writing in the *Lancet*, Dr D. R. Rosseinsky and Dr P. G. Hall proposed, I think seriously, the theory that PMS was part of a phase of deliberately pro-grammed female hostility, built in by evolutionary forces and designed to discourage the male from wasting his sexual energies at a time when conception would not be possible.[11] The thwarted male would presumably turn to more responsive and receptive females, whose tempers were not hormonally dis-turbed, and whose ovulatory cycles were favourable to fertili-zation.

It is not a theory likely to convince many doctors or appeal to many women, and it certainly does not fit in with the more widely accepted concept of the importance of pair-bonding – the system by which two human beings are first attracted to each other and later kept together. It seems far more likely, if evolution is to be dragged in at all, that the human female is still only in the process of adaptation to the peculiarly human system of monthly menstruation. It is probably that menstrua-tion itself is not really natural and that initially the human female was designed to become pregnant on first ovulation, breast-feed each offspring for two years and then become pregnant again. With this system she would never really suffer from menstruation and menstrual problems, so that PMS may be simply an adverse response to hormonal fluctuations not experienced by our primate ancestors.

In view of the fact that it may take evolution a few more million years to get the faulty mechanism ironed out, it is just as well that research into this common and long-neglected problem is beginning to provide answers by treating the root causes.

It has been immensely satisfying, as it was when reporting on HRT for the menopause, to be able to report the successful outcome of the St Thomas's trials and generally to alert women to the existence now of various new ways of dealing with PMS. Again as with the menopause, each article, radio or television item on PMS has brought a flood of letters. Many of these women have now been helped and more and more are receiving appropriate hormonal treatment direct from their GPs. Postgraduate courses on PMS are starting to proliferate as they did on the menopause and HRT; medical literature also carries reports of the new work. The controlled trials which are needed before any treatment gains widespread acceptance are already under way.

Phone-ins on both HRT and PMS are producing more and more response on PMS. At one time the menopause problems always dominated but now the questions divide equally between the two. The message is certainly spreading at the lay level, but it is noticeable also that seminars and meetings are more and more combining the two subjects at medical level; this is a good thing, as between them they cover the whole age-range at least from puberty upwards, and this seems to be increasing the response from doctors and para-medical workers such as nurses, health visitors, etc.

Talking on HRT, it was always important to try and introduce some humour and it is the same now with PMS. I was delighted to find Dr T. C. G. Smith, one of our best medical communicators, at a recent seminar drawing a harrowing picture of the sheik facing his harem of women, not only all menstruating at the same time, due to their communal living, but *all* with PMS at the same time!

It's certainly worth recording here the surge of interest in PMS, reflected by attendances and by the rapidly changing attitude of doctors toward the problem. You may find even if your own doctor only prescribed diuretic or pain-killers when you consulted him a year or so ago, he may well have changed his views now and be prepared to try newer methods.

Perhaps the final word on the subject should come from

Rosalynd Cook, one of the first women to write to me for help and one of those taking part in the original St Thomas's study. Rosalynd, who is thirty-one now, hit trouble after the birth of her baby, suffering severe depression, sore breasts and a weight gain of around seven pounds. A biology teacher with scientific training, she set out to keep a record of her symptoms and their time of onset, soon establishing that it all started precisely ten days before menstruation. She told me:

Valium and sleeping tablets were prescribed but life had become terribly difficult for us as a family and we struggled on for three years, with me having only quite a short time each month when I really felt anything like normal. I can only say now after hormonal treatment that things are really looking up. It's marvellous to feel well and energetic again and I have been able to get back to teaching four days a week as well as enjoying my home and family life. I know so many other women who suffer in the same way and I feel I want them all to realize they don't have to go on putting up with PMS – the treatment is there if they will just make the effort to get it.

4. Conception

In theory, at this point we should be content with a short, factual account of conception and what happens when a male sperm meets, penetrates and fertilizes a female egg. That is all that is actually needed to understand how life begins and how modern contraceptive techniques work by blocking the normal mechanisms.

In practice, however, it's an irresistible temptation to share something of the awe and wonder invoked by a process which, through a form of genetic roulette, shuffles together two sets of chromosomes and genes and, starting from a single cell, nine months later delivers a new and unique human being, made up of twenty-six trillion highly organized and specialized cells.

It's no wonder that the primitive mind had to try to explain creation and new life in terms of some sort of miraculous supernatural involvement. The real truth of natural evolvement is even more incredible, with the genetic mix, match and mutation working through the generations, for adaptation and survival – a slow, painful progress that has brought us from floundering in primeval mud to walking upright, discovering fire, inventing the wheel and finally soaring out toward the stars.

Heredity

Whatever the potential for humanity as a whole, the potential for each human being as an individual is laid down at the moment of conception, written and coded on pairs of genes, which are strung like beads on the twenty-three pairs of chromosomes contained in each cell of the body.

The chromosomes are actually visible under the microscope and are made up of connected strands of the chemical DNA (deoxyribonucleic acid) which forms the genes, the smallest unit of information. These genes control things like eye colour, nose shape, height and so on, with half of them coming from the father through the male sperm and half from the mother contained in the female egg. In addition to physical characteristics genes also determine potential intelligence, temperament and special abilities, such as skill in art, music or sport, all of which can be inherited just as much as dark eyes or curly hair.

The word 'potential' is necessary in this context, however, because environment can later modify, diminish or reinforce heredity. Just as full physical potential may not be realized if a child is undernourished or neglected, so also the potential for intelligence or musical ability may never be fully realized without opportunity, encouragement, education and training.

Exact replicas of all the chromosomes and all the genes go into every cell as they divide and form, but while some genes have work to do in every part of the body, others only go into action if they are in a cell where their special craft is needed, to make pigment for instance, or to form bones, or transmit messages.

Sex-determination

The most fundamental set of directions transmitted by the chromosomes and genes is the one determining our sex. Among our twenty-three pairs of chromosomes each of us has one special pair of sex chromosomes. In women these are both of one type, called X, and together form the female XX combination. In men, however, there are two kinds – the same familiar X type and another smaller Y type – which together give the male XY formation. The different shapes of the two types of chromosomes can be clearly distinguished under a microscope.

In just one special type of cell, the mature sex cell (the egg of the female and the sperm of the male), instead of twenty-three *pairs* of chromosomes as in all other cells, there are only twenty-three *single* chromosomes bearing *single* genes. This means that when the sperm is ejaculated from the male penis during intercourse and one of the millions of sperm manages to penetrate and fertilize the female egg, the genetic contributions from each parent come together, joining up once again to form twenty-three *pairs* of chromosomes. The genes pair off once more, but in a new alignment, to form a new blueprint for a new person.

So it is the father who actually determines the sex of the baby. If a Y sperm wins the procreation race to penetrate and fertilize the female egg, which already contains its own X chromosome, this XY combination produces a boy. If an X sperm reaches the egg first, the XX combination proceeds to order up and form a girl.

Sex ratio of boys and girls

Although variations occur in different parts of the world, between 104 and 107 boys are born for every 100 girls in most countries. In the past, more males died of disease and injury at all stages of life, leaving a surplus of females from adolescence onwards. Recently this has changed. Medical advances have now reduced early male deaths and there is now a surplus of men, at least until early middle age, when the greater suscepti-bility of men to coronary attacks begins to change the balance. In Great Britain there are some 103 males to every 100 females between the ages of fifteen and forty-nine, whereas in the past there were only about 92.

Doctors now know that the number of males to females is even higher in the earlier stages of pregnancy than it is at birth. This is because nature's own system of quality control comes into play with large numbers of spontaneous abortions taking place, often because of some deformity or bad genetic traits. For every 100 females aborted in this way there are some 135 males. From this known fact, it has to be assumed that more male sperm win the procreation race in the first instance – and in many ways this is probably logical as they are smaller and have longer tails which seems to help them to swim somewhat faster. On the other hand, while the male Y-type sperm is what someone called a 'fast and flashy' performer in the short run, it is the female sperm which has more staying power and is more robust. This sort of knowledge is now being used in efforts to predetermine the sex of a child.

Influencing sex at conception

All over the world research is going on to find a method of influencing sex at conception, so that there is at least an increased chance of having a baby of the particular sex you want.

One of the men who has done a great deal of work on this is a New York obstetrician, Landrum Shettles, who has made a special study of human eggs and sperm for over forty years. His recommendations and methods for influencing sex at conception are controversial, but are now attracting attention in this country too, where similar work is also under way. At the simplest level Dr Shettles believes that any conditions which make conception easier favour a male baby. Conditions which make conception harder favour the tougher, hardier female sperm.

His guidelines for couples wanting a girl are to have intercourse as desired until two days before ovulation and then stop for a week. This works on the theory that female sperm can usually survive the waiting period until the egg emerges from the ovary, while the less robust male sperms are more likely to die off.

There is support for the theory that the timing factor is crucial.[12] Dr William James, Associate Research Fellow at University College, London, and an acknowledged expert on this subject, told me:

My own work certainly confirms that timing is the key factor, but it's also indisputable that more boys are born both during and immediately after wars. I believe this is related to the higher incidence of intercourse, what you might term the *rate* of intercourse, which seems to favour conception by the male sperm. Obviously servicemen in wartime and on short leave or returning after long separation at the end of hostilities will be more sexually active. The same applies, of course, during early months of marriage and again it has been shown that a higher proportion of boys are born to women who conceive within eighteen months of marriage.

Dr Shettles also believes that, to favour conception of a girl, a woman should use an acid douche immediately before intercourse – two tablespoons of white vinegar in a quart of water is his simple home-made recipe. This is supposed to help because female sperm are known to thrive in an acid environment which is hostile to the male sperm. So, for the same reason, Shettles suggests any woman wanting a girl baby should refrain from actual orgasm, as this produces alkaline fluids favourable to male sperm. He also believes ejaculation of sperm only just inside the vagina favours a girl rather than deep penetration, on the theory that if the short race goes to the swift male sperm, the longer race is more likely to go to the competitor with most stamina – in this case the tougher female sperm.

For those prepared to try out the Shettles theory, exactly the opposite tactics are supposed to be used to favour conception of a boy. Most importantly, the couple should refrain from intercourse until the actual day of ovulation is expected. The woman should try to achieve orgasm and so provide the alkaline fast track favouring the fast-swimming male sperm. For the same reason an alkaline douche is recommended before inter-course. The recipe for this is equally homely: two tablespoons of baking soda fully dissolved in a quart of water. Obviously, deep penetration is also desirable, allowing the shorter race to favour the fast but less enduring male sperm.

In America Dr Shettles claimed on 80 per cent success rate for his combined systems, with some 200 women taking part in his experiments. It is only fair to point out that experts in this country are extremely sceptical and that doctors here are very much opposed on principle to methods and treatments which involve douching.

Douching is seen by most British doctors as a peculiarly American and unnecessary obsession with cleanliness since the vagina, as already mentioned, cleans itself producing a lactic acid designed specifically for the job. Douches dilute or wash this acid out, and they can also be a source of infection in them-selves, particularly if they reach the opening to the cervix. There is also the hazard of air-bubbles or of the liquid being too hot and damage being done to the lining of the vagina.

Nevertheless, Dr Shettles's acid–alkaline theory has already been followed up in Great Britain, and one doctor has even gone to the length of patenting a 'do-it-yourself' child selection kit. Dr John Pollard, a Manchester consultant anaesthetist, was reported in the lay press as planning to market a gelatine-based compound to control acid levels, claiming that it should greatly increase the chance of conceiving a baby of the desired sex. Under the appropriate name, Choice, it has yet to be proven effective for humans and only ten women in this country have so far tried it. But Dr Pollard does admit: 'There still has to be careful, lengthy and unhurried research applicable to any new product and rightly so. Double blind trials are now planned and I would hope for market availability in five years.'

Meanwhile the ingenious Dr Shettles has invented a screening device designed to aid conception of boys. This will permit the smaller-headed male sperm to pass through more easily than the larger-headed female ones. Placed like a diaphragm across the entrance of the cervix, Dr Shettle insists it does not discourage the determined sperm, which he describes as 'wild to get into the mucus of the cervix', but it does tend to filter out the female sperm. In twenty-eight tests, the sperms that got through were 89 to 97 per cent male, but it still has to be shown whether, after the struggle, they retain the capacity to fertilize the egg.

Other methods, of course, apply for anyone prepared to consider artificial insemination, where various means of separating sperm into male and female batches have been tried with varying success. Centrifuging (spinning at high speeds) is supposed to cause the heavier ones (usually female) to end up at the bottom but some scientists feel the process might also cause risk of chromosomal damage.

Electrical separation, based on the fact that male and female sperm have different electrical charges, has also been tried in Russia and in the US. Male sperm drift to a negative pole and female to a positive pole. By making sperm pass through a sticky substance carrying an electric charge, one biochemist in America in 1973 achieved progeny in animals that was up to 95 per cent female, because the male sperm stuck to the resin. To achieve males instead of females, it is possible simply to wash the male sperm free from the resin.

Obviously most of the research and most of these methods are directed toward animal rather than human breeding. It is fascinating that the simple peasants of India elect to bring their cattle at dusk for artificial insemination, after the can of sperm has been standing all day. The process of the heavier female sperm tending to sink means that by drawing fluid from the top there is a greater chance of male sperm to produce the male animals they want.

It really remains to be seen whether successful predetermination of sex for human babies is achieved. If so, it will probably be through some adaptation of these methods and not through such old wives' tales as conceiving in June favouring boys or foggy weather being linked to conception of girls. One pea-soup fog in London in 1954 was supposed to be responsible for the very high ratio of female babies reported by London hospitals nine months later. It is quite amazing that people could ever believe this; though, as our weather gets blamed for most things, perhaps we should not be altogether surprised.

Methods and technology, perfectly acceptable for agriculture and animals, must often be far more dubious when applied to humans. So it is not entirely a question of whether eventually a way of effectively influencing the sex of our children could be found but whether it *should* be found, and if so, whether it should be widely used.

A survey done in America among woman showed only 39 per cent of them in favour of the idea, but there could well be higher interest among men. Certainly two-thirds of couples questioned in another study had a definite preference for the sex of their child, with 90 per cent wanting the firstborn to be a boy. And one can well understand a couple with perhaps three daughters rather desperately wanting a boy fourth time round; or a couple with all boys being grateful for any method which increased the chances for a longed-for daughter.

There are understandable and human reasons in favour of effective sex-control technology, the rather grand term coined for what is still rather hit-and-miss theory at the moment.

But a sound medical argument would certainly lie in the ability to choose the sex of a baby deliberately to avoid the risk of having some genetic sex-linked disease. Haemophilia, muscular dystrophy and night-blindness, for example, are carried by females but usually only afflict males.

Again, sex-control technology, once perfected, could be important to countries like India, where population control is vital if real progress is to be made and living standards raised.

At the moment, wherever there is great poverty, there is also, ironically, resistance to birth control, simply because people go on having children in the hope of achieving enough sons to support them in old age. With sex control, once an adequate number of boys was achieved, birth control would be more attractive.

The few surveys that have been done suggest that in the developed world there would also be a swing toward more boy babies, but probably to around 60 per cent only. Allowing for accidental conceptions, failure of sex-control techniques and the greater chance of boy babies dying, Vance Packard, author of the fascinating book, *The People Shapers*, estimates the male–female ratio would settle down to around 55 males to 45 females. Even that would considerably change the situation for women, giving them what he terms 'a chooser's market'. But he also believes it could give us a tougher and presumably even more violent world, quoting the sociologist, Amitai Etzioni, who believes that criminality would increase and that the world would suffer from the reduction of the civilizing effect he attributes to women, with their greater interest in cultural activities.

Like so many of the technological advances either already with us or just around the corner, predetermination of sex could well solve old problems for the individual but pose new problems for society.

Sexual differentiation

Whatever sex we are ultimately destined to be, a surprising fact is that we all actually start out as bisexual, equipped with rudimentary organs and ducts for both sexes and capable of development in either direction.

It is only during the fourth month of life in the womb that nature's computer irrevocably switches the foetus along a single-sex road. If programmed by an XY chromosome, the male organs and ducts develop or, if by an XX chromosome, the female organs; in both cases, the other structures are left untouched and undeveloped.

Once this sexual differentiation has begun, the sex hormones secreted by the growing male testes or the female ovaries take over and continue to govern the direction of development both before birth and again later at puberty.

As adults, the reminders of our bisexual beginnings are still apparent in the non-functioning nipples of the man, and the clitoris of the woman which is really only the undeveloped penis. Rather disconcertingly, women also have all the hair follicles present for a full beard and moustache, but happily these normally lie dormant. Occasionally after the menopause, when oestrogen – the main female hormone – declines, there is sufficient swing toward the male hormone, testosterone, to trigger some hair growth on face and even chest, which can be distressing. Prompt hormone treatment can help this by restoring the female balance, but HRT used in good time is even more effective in preventing it.

We are so conditioned to think of ourselves in the human race as either totally female or totally male, with our roles and responses clearly defined according to gender, that it is perhaps a good thing to recognize that there is a spectrum of sexuality. Each of us produces some hormones of the other sex. Men produce small amounts of oestrogen and women produce small amounts of testosterone. There is the very male male at one end of the spectrum and the very female female at the other, but in between some women have all the drive and enterprise traditionally associated with the male, while some men have the compassion and sensitivity more associated with the female. These differences cannot usually be tied in directly with hormone levels in adult life, but certainly the balance can be crucial to physical development and most especially before birth, when the developing foetus is particularly vulnerable.

As mentioned earlier the female is now known to be the basic sex and, left to itself, every foetus would turn toward the female. Only the powerful and continuous intervention of the male sex hormone effects the differentiation which results in a boy.

Happily, for most of us nature's controlling computer works correctly, but in just a few cases something goes wrong and too much oestrogen reaching a male foetus results in feminization, while too much testosterone reaching a female foetus produces the masculinization of a girl.

In the past, when a busy midwife or doctor might never before have seen a case of enlarged clitoris or poorly developed male genitalia, it was sometimes possible for the wrong sex to be assigned and the child to be registered and brought up in the wrong gender. The tragedy was usually only then discovered at puberty, when the child brought up as a girl failed to develop breasts and to menstruate or the child brought up as a boy proceeded to do both. The shock for everyone concerned must have been appalling, and at that stage and in those days little could be done to undo either the physical or psychological damage.

Once again we can be grateful that we live in an age when modern medicine can prevent such tragedies. Today, if there is the slightest suspicion of sexual ambiguity, at birth, a simple test will establish the real sex. A few cells are taken from inside the mouth, stained and viewed under the microscope. In female cells there is a special content (chromatin) which this process shows up, called the Barr body, after the researcher who discovered it. So the presence of a Barr body in the nucleus indicates a female and its absence, a male. This is known as the 'nuclear' sex and, if it is found to contradict the gender of the predominant physical characteristics, then fuller investigation must be done to establish the actual chromosome constitution. Corrective hormone treatment and surgery, if necessary, can then be undertaken at the appropriate time.

This sort of physical intersex, as it is called, is extremely rare and proven hormonal or chromosomal defects clearly cause it. But what some people see as *psychological* intersex, usually blamed on upbringing and childhood experience, may also eventually prove to have its roots in abnormal hormone influences *before* birth. This may involve the 4 per cent of men and women who have sexual drive toward their own sex, usually called homosexuality in the male and lesbianism in a woman. But it also includes the rare and more tragic transsexuals who from a very young age are totally convinced they belong to the opposite sex and are simply trapped in the wrong body. Neither psychotherapy nor the drastic forms of aversion therapy that have been tried have succeeded in overcoming the problem. With the true transsexual the conviction is so deep and the drive so strong that they endeavour to dress and live in the desired sex, often helped in the first instance by appropriate hormone treatment. If they manage in this way to achieve a more tolerable life, they usually go on to ask for the extensive and painful surgery which will in their view take them nearer to their longed-for gender. At best, it usually remains a twilight half-life, always precarious and with formal marriage impossible. While all other documentation can be changed, under our existing laws the birth certificate cannot and, as marriage is essentially a contract between a man and a women, any form of ceremony involving two people of the same sex has no legal standing, despite any hormonal or surgical intervention.

If I have given almost too much space to what is really only a rare problem, it is because I feel knowing something about it should help us all to be more understanding. Dr C. M. Armstrong of Newcastle-upon-Tyne, one of the leading authorities on intersex problems, pointed out to me:

> Primitive human instinct is to reject the deviant, but the more civilized society becomes and the more we understand the underlying causes, the more we should accept the spectrum of sexuality in all its variety. We should be thankful when we and our children fall within the normal range, and feel only compassion toward the minority, who through no fault of their own, are faced with the distressing problems of living in our society and somehow coping with their own different sexuality in *our* world.

Implantation for growth

Thankfully for the great majority of the human race, nature's computer works correctly and normal development starts immediately after a sperm has penetrated the shell of the egg. The sperm's tail is stuck in the soft shell and drops off, leaving the sperm head containing the vital nucleus with its twenty-three chromosomes, inside the female egg.

Once the female cell with its own twenty-three chromosomes recognizes that it is now equipped with the full complement of genetic information necessary to make a new individual, it starts to divide – first into two identical cells, then four, then again, doubling each time. These divisions take place outside the womb during the three days that it takes the fertilized egg to move along the oviduct (fallopian tube) to the womb. Once inside the uterus the still-growing mass of cells separates into two parts. One is the outer shell of cells which will form the placenta, the surrounding spongy substance through which nourishment passes from mother to baby during pregnancy. The other cells, the inner group, will form the embryo. Very soon after this the original outer shell of the egg dissolves and the fertilized egg (officially called at this stage a blastocyst, which seems a very unprepossessing name) plants itself in the soft lining of the womb.

Nine days after fertilization, and when it is still only the size of a pin-head, the tiny embryo should be deeply implanted and growing rapidly. The placenta, of course, grows too and the space between the egg and the placenta becomes lined with special membranes containing protective shock-absorbing fluid. In medical language this is called the amniotic sac and the waters are known as amniotic fluid. The placenta and the embryo (officially called the foetus from the eighth week of pregnancy) work together with the placenta, acting as lungs, liver and kidney for the foetus. Oxygen is carried to it, and waste products taken away, by the mother's blood, to reduce the work the tiny growing liver and kidneys need to do. The foetus and placenta also combine to produce various hormones vital to maintain the pregnancy.

The mother's blood does not mix with the blood of the foetus but washes round the placental cells which, like a sponge, allow nourishment and oxygen to pass through into tiny blood vessels inside the placenta. These join up then into larger vessels running through the umbilical cord, the tube which links the growing baby to the placenta.

Later, in Chapter 9, we can follow the marvellous process to its conclusion, the birth of a new life. But such a life must be part of a planned and wanted family. For many women and for many reasons there are times when a baby is not wanted. So now we must look at contraceptive techniques, how they work, their reliability, their safety, their advantages and their drawbacks. At least today there is a wide choice and a free family planning service.

5. Contraception

If I had to pick out one area of medicine which has brought most benefit to the individual woman and to society as a whole, it would have to be modern contraception.

Freedom to plan your family, to have only *wanted* children, is fundamental to their happiness and to yours. Modern, fully effective contraception is also essential to women achieving equality in jobs and careers, and in selection for training and promotion.

Family planning has been described as 'preventive medicine *par excellence*', and certainly the prevention of unwanted births prevents in turn a great many social and human ills.

Of Britain's population (fifty-four million), there are ten and a half million women in the fertile age range. Of these, an estimated eight million are believed to be sexually active and at risk of pregnancy. Normally any young fertile woman with the opportunity to conceive has a 60 per cent chance of becoming pregnant in any one month. In some cases, of course, there can be special problems, and even reading about contraception must be irritating to women or couples faced with infertility. But at least there is a great deal of hopeful new work in that area, and it is described in the next chapter.

But in general, *over*-fertility is the problem, and in our over-populated world family planning is a sound investment. Even free family planning for all who want it actually represents a considerable long-term saving to the tax-payer. The government has recognized this in making the service now free under the National Health, though at the time of writing there are still a few anomalies.

It seems strange, for instance, that while the widely used male contraceptive, the sheath or condom, can be freely pre-scribed in family planning clinics, it still *cannot* be prescribed by a GP.

When Dr David Owen was Minister of State for Health he estimated that by 1978–9 the total cost of a free comprehensive family planning service would be around £50 million. But he also pointed out that the cost, so often discounted, of any one birth to the public funds is about £3400, so that the number of unwanted births only had to be reduced by 15000 to cover this cost. With yearly figures running at 55000 illegitimate births, 45000 conceptions before marriage and 100000 abortions, there could be little argument about the need for free and fuller birth control services.

In their evidence to the Royal Commission on the NHS in the autumn of 1977, the Family Planning Association gave the up-to-date figure for unwanted pregnancies in the UK as 200000 a year, 20000 of which were illegitimate births to women under twenty. They also made a strong point regarding the anomalies I have mentioned, asking for them to be investigated and stating that about two and a half million couples in the UK use the sheath, a considerable number against which to discriminate by forbidding GP prescription. They also urged on economic grounds more use of clinic services for birth control, particularly for the Pill, which costs between £6 and £7 a year for a clinic patient but £9 a year under a GP.

Removal of the prudish and hypocritical ban on advertising of family planning on television, public transport and in certain journals and newspapers would do a great deal to help to get accurate information across. It's absurd in an age when sex itself is used as the basis of so much commercial advertising and presented often so blatantly on our screens, for objections to be raised to responsible advertising of measures which at least help to prevent the disasters unwanted pregnancies can involve. About the time one leading newspaper refused Health Education advertisements to increase contraceptive awareness, it was publishing articles on 'Sex secrets of the local stud', 'How to tell if she's a virgin' and 'Playing the field'. Despite this they had the nerve to reject the contraceptive material on the ground that 'it was in poor taste'.

More clinics, more domiciliary services and a better display by chemists of local clinic addresses would all encourage more people to take advantage of the free service and help to remove lingering embarrassment about what, in this age, in an over-populated world, should be a social duty if we care about the future for our children.

Obviously, in some cases, religious objections enter into the picture. More and more educated Catholics are opting for freedom of conscience and decision and using the Pill, albeit sometimes under the euphemism of menstrual regulator instead of contraceptive – the result is the same. Others, often those least able to cope with the burden of repeated pregnancies and large families crammed into poor housing, submit to the Pope's ruling and their priests' admonitions. While it's only right to respect deeply held beliefs, the whole position now does appear totally illogical.

From the time the Catholic Church accepted that the rhythm method of birth control was permissible, it also accepted that sexual intercourse could be for something other than procreation. With this basic change of stance, it now seems absurd to insist that menstrual charts, basal temperatures, thermometers, and sex according to the calendar rather than desire, is somehow more natural than the Pill which, after all, works by adjusting natural hormone levels and allows expression of natural feelings at a natural time.

The full consequences of all this is not only felt in the individual families – marriages under stress from attempts at abstinence and mothers whose health is broken by too much childbearing – but it is felt throughout the world in the failure of efforts to bring rational family planning to the poorer Catholic countries – in particular in Spain, Portugal and South America. Without population control there is no hope of raising standards of living. It also has the far worse effect from the Catholic Church's point of view of driving good Catholic women in desperation to seek abortion. It is significant that most of the women coming to Britain for abortion from Europe are from the Catholic countries of Spain, Portugal, Italy and Eire.

All one should ask for is that every woman has the choice of contraception *if* she wants it, and, with the advice of her doctor or family planning clinic, the method best suited to her needs. So let us consider the possibilities already available, their advantages, disadvantages, and relative effectiveness.

Coitus interruptus

Withdrawal of the penis from the vagina just before ejaculation of sperm in an effort to avoid pregnancy is the oldest and most widely used method. It depends very much on the man being able to recognize the crucial moment and having the self-control to pull out. It's not only a very uncertain method with a high risk of pregnancy – the failure rate has been estimated at 25 per cent over a twelve-month period – but it also leaves the woman with pelvic discomfort, if she had been stimulated but not relieved. It diminishes the pleasure of the man, too, forcing him to withdraw at the very moment when he most wants even deeper penetration. Fortunately now there are better methods.

The rhythm method

It is doubtful whether this qualifies as a better method, as the failure rate is even higher, at 30 per cent over twelve months. It is based on avoiding intercourse on the days when the woman is calculated to be at her most fertile. Ovulation takes place usually thirteen to fifteen days before the first day of the next menstrual period and sperm can only survive for about seventy-two hours in the genital tract. So if the couple abstain from coitus for three days on each side of the supposed time of ovulation, in theory pregnancy should not occur. Unfortunately, as the failure rate indicates, ovulation can occur at other times in the cycle, sometimes under the spur of special emotion or stress. To overcome this, attempts are made to pinpoint ovulation by noting the rise of temperature which indicates its onset. But if intercourse has taken place the day before the rise is noted, the sperm may well still be active when ovulation occurs. Perhaps the only really safe 'safe' period is during actual menstruation; and although somewhat messy, it can often be a time when women experience an increase in sexual desire.

Douching

This is only listed because many women *believe* it is a method of contraception to douche immediately after intercourse. In fact it is useless, merely washing out the sperm left in the vagina but doing nothing about the thousands which will have entered the cervix already. It is also pretty destructive of any sexual relationship for one partner to leap out of bed just at the moment when relaxation together should complete the pleasure.

Chemical methods

There are various preparations in the forms of jellies, foams and creams, all containing chemicals which will kill any sperm in contact with them for long enough. They are usually introduced high into the vagina with a tube and plunger just prior to intercourse, but used alone they are a poor method of protection, with a failure rate, similar to the rhythm method, amounting to 30 per cent. They can, however, be a valuable addition to the efficiency of the vaginal cap or diaphragm.

The diaphragm or cap

This consists of a thin rubber dome which has a coiled spring in the rim and is made in various sizes. In the first instance, to ensure the right size, it must be fitted by a doctor or family planning specialist. The woman is then taught to smear the anti-sperm jelly or cream around the rim of the cap and insert it herself, by squeezing and pushing it up into position and then releasing it to regain its shape and cover the cervix. It should normally be inserted routinely every night, then removed and washed the next morning or not less than six hours *after* coitus. Used correctly, it is good protection against pregnancy (and sound evidence also suggests against cervical cancer) while not affecting the pleasure for either partner. But it does require intelligence and a certain dexterity to use it properly. The failure rate when used in conjunction with a chemical agent is only 10 per cent. A woman who has had a baby since having her diaphragm first fitted may well find she needs a larger size next time round.

The condom or sheath

This also works on the barrier principle to prevent sperm

reaching the cervix, but it involves covering the penis, usually after erection, which some men and their partners may find disconcerting. For maximum safety the condom should be put on before the penis is even inserted into the vagina. Delaying the application until just before orgasm will often result in pregnancy, as there can be seepage of sperm on occasion before actual orgasm. Accidents can also happen if the sheath is not removed very carefully or if it tears. Despite the drawbacks the failure rate is only 15 per cent and it is a widely practised method, largely because the fine latex rubber now used does not interfere with sensation, and because of easy availability over the chemist's counter and from machines. It is a method which has been used since Roman times and it has the virtue of protecting against VD; in many armies condoms became virtually general issue to soldiers thought to be at risk from contact with prostitutes. For a woman it also offers protection against transmission of very common infections like monilia and trichomonas, which will be discussed later.

The IUD (intra-uterine device)

Intra-uterine means 'inside the womb' and the IUD is a small device, usually between one and two inches in length. It is small, flat, flexible and comes in varying shapes. Loops and coils in plastic, sometimes covered with copper, are most commonly used today.

They say there is nothing new under the sun, which is a slight exaggeration, but certainly the IUD in one form or another has been known since Biblical times. Arab camel drivers used to introduce a small stone the size of a pea into the uterus of their female camels before a long desert journey to ensure they did not become pregnant.

But the real breakthrough came in modern times with the development of polythene, a plastic which regains its shape after stretching, does not irritate the tissues, can be made free from germs and is *cheap*. This is vitally important if birth control is ever to become widespread in the developing countries where it is most needed.

There are advantages other than cheapness. Once fitted the loop or coil can be left in place for several years. One type,

called the Copper 7, should be replaced every two years. Otherwise, after a first check-up between six and twelve weeks after
fitting, a yearly check is all that is normally required. The
woman herself can ensure that the device has not been expelled,
something which occasionally happens. For this reason a little
string is fitted to the I U D which can be easily felt in the vagina.
If the string cannot be detected, then a visit to the doctor is indicated. But the failure rate is very low indeed, only 3 per cent,
which is approaching the figure for the progestogen-only pill
(one of the types of contraceptive pill).

Before an I U D is fitted, the doctor will normally check to
make sure the uterus is normal, and that there is no possibility
of a pregnancy already in progress. For the woman who has
already had a child, fitting the I U D should not be painful. For
the woman who has not, there may be slight discomfort and
some doctors offer pain-killers or valium. After the fitting many
women experience cramp-like pain rather like that sometimes
associated with a period, but it does not last long and soluble
aspirin or a hot water bottle helps. In just a few cases there can
be more serious complications such as pelvic inflammation and,
very rarely, actual perforation of the womb. But for most
women, especially those who have had several children, the
I U D is often an excellent method. Intercourse is safe immediately after fitting and the device does not interfere in any way
either with this or with periods, though the first few may be
heavier than usual and, just occasionally, at first there is a little
bleeding between periods. But things soon settle back to normal.
If they do not, then you must consult your doctor. It is estimated
that for one woman in five, the I U D is not totally satisfactory.

If you want a baby the I U D is simply removed, but this
must be done by your doctor or at your family planning clinic.
The I U D should also be removed if by any chance pregnancy
does occur but, as the statistics show, this is most unlikely.

The main reason for some women finding the I U D unacceptable has been heavier periods. A new form of I U D which contains the female hormone, progesterone, and is called a 'progestasert' has recently been used to try and counteract this. It
has proved to reduce the amount of menstrual bleeding but not
the duration, and the fact that it has to be changed every
eighteen months is a distinct disadvantage. On the other hand,

there is some evidence that the progestasert is less often expelled spontaneously than other devices; this may be due to what doctors term the 'quieting' effect that the slow release of progesterone is believed to have on the uterus.

How the IUD works

Women are usually more concerned that a birth control method works and is safe than with why it works or how it works. But the IUD poses a rather different situation, at least for the Catholic woman or Catholic doctor, as there has been mounting suspicion over a long period that it functions not so much as a true contraceptive but as an abortifacient, actually preventing implantation of the already fertilized egg and in some way bringing about its destruction.

Work reported by the World Health Organization as far back as 1966 confirmed that an IUD did not disturb the menstrual cycle, ovulation, movement of sperm or egg through the fallopian tubes, or even fertilization. Fertilized eggs have frequently been recovered from the fallopian tubes of women fitted with IUDs.

Then in 1975, at the Universidad Católica de Chile in Santiago, Dr Croxatto managed to show that while eggs could be recovered from the fallopian tubes in women with or without a uterine device, no eggs or embryos could be recovered from the actual womb of women fitted with an IUD. So what was happening to them? Were they failing to enter the uterus? Were they entering but being expelled very rapidly? Or were they being destroyed in some way in the uterus as they tried to implant?

The work in Chile was carried out on women who came to hospital for sterilization, which is about the only ethical source for research and embryo recovery in human females, but of course limits the recovery techniques which can be used.

So instead, as so often, the scientists had to follow up and study the problem further in animals. Fortunately, although it's perhaps not very flattering, the female Rhesus monkey offers a close and valid comparison to the human female, at least in reproductive matters. They also have a twenty-eight-day cycle and ovulate between days twelve and fifteen, as does the average woman, and they also fail to conceive when fitted with an IUD.

It was only in 1977 that a team at Birmingham University Medical School came up with real proof that the IUD was causing destruction of actual tiny embryos. The researchers had already devised a method of flushing out the uterus, which proved to yield pre-implantation embryos in 50 per cent of mated female monkeys *not* fitted with an IUD.

The monkeys from whom embryos had been recovered in this way were then fitted with the coil and, after two successive cycles, mated again. When they were flushed, as before, between days fifteen and twenty of the cycle, far fewer embryos were recovered and they were *all abnormal, degenerating and under attack from large numbers of white blood cells* (part of the body's immune mechanism designed to attack and destroy invaders).[13]

Dr Peter Hurst, who carried out the Birmingham research, commented:

It had been suspected that the IUDs probably worked by acting as a foreign body and setting up a hostile inflammatory reaction which prevents implantation. We certainly proved it works that way in Rhesus monkeys, and in conjunction with the work of the World Health Organization and Dr Croxatto, I think we must assume the same mechanism at work in humans.

The significance of these findings lies in the effect on Roman Catholic doctors who oppose abortion, but have until now been prepared to fit IUDs.

The new evidence that IUDs work by destroying the developing embryo was widely reported in the medical and lay press and, in particular, on 30 September 1977, in *General Practitioner*, a special newspaper sent to all family doctors. The anti-abortion lobby has always argued that the ovum or egg acquires 'uniquely human potential' and therefore human rights from the moment of fertilization, and so it is totally inconsistent for doctors like Margaret White to go on thundering against abortion while continuing to fit IUDs. And it is even more inconsistent for doctors to fit the IUD, almost certainly causing death of early embryos, while refusing to use the Pill, which works by the truly contraceptive technique of preventing fertilization from ever taking place.

The contraceptive pill

Most of us talk about the contraceptive pill as if there was just one type. In fact there are about twenty-seven different brands, containing different kinds, doses and combinations of female hormones. But they all work by rather cleverly fooling the body: they raise the female hormone levels as in pregnancy and, as with a true pregnancy, a signal is received by the pituitary gland which controls the whole process and no further ovulation takes place.

I suppose that in any definitive history of the world, the year 1957 would have to go down as the beginning of the Age of the Pill. It had been known for some time that small doses of the female hormone oestrogen given from the end of menstruation could prevent ovulation, but unfortunately the menstrual period following was prolonged with a further phase of unacceptable spotting. It was also known that injections of the second female hormone each day for six days alongside the oestrogen just prior to the next menstrual cycle ensured a much more normal period. Daily injections, of course, are not practical and so the search was well and truly on to find some substitute for progesterone which would work but could be taken by mouth.

It was Dr Pincus, an American scientist, who came up with the answer. He found that the Mexican yam, a vegetable a bit like a potato, yielded a substance with a progesterone-like action even when taken orally. It was called a 'gestagen' and all the refinements and developments since are called 'progestogens'. By 1957 two years' trials on human volunteers had proved both effective and safe. The combination of hormones taken by mouth became known as the oral contraceptive and later more colloquially as just the Pill. It soon became widely used because it had great advantages, particularly in the more affluent, developed countries.

It is virtually 100 per cent effective. The failure rate on this combined pill is only 0·25 per cent, a quarter of one per cent. It is easy to take, no privacy is needed, it allows spontaneous love-making at any time and, as an added bonus for many women, it regulates periods and even reduces menstrual loss and pain. It also allows women (in cooperation with their doctors) to adjust their periods occasionally to fit in with holidays and honeymoons.

C

With wider usage and greater experience, it was found possible to reduce considerably the amount of both sex hormones without reducing the effectiveness and the new family of pills all belong to this low-dosage category.

There are three main types of the Pill, with many minor variations within each type. First there is the ordinary combined pill which we have been describing; secondly, there is what is termed the 'sequential' type no longer used in Britain. Here oestrogen is given in the first part of the cycle and the progestogen only added in the later part, more closely simulating the natural hormone pattern.

To make it all as simple as possible, many drug companies produced special packs with the days of the cycle numbered and sometimes even the days of the week named. This has also been done with the ordinary combined pill. With the sequential pill it was decided to try a twenty-eight-day continuous pill-taking cycle, although the pill doses during the last seven days contained only sugar or very minute doses of hormone so that menstruation still took place. This type of sequential pill is not quite as effective as the ordinary combined pill; it has a 2 per cent failure rate.

The third type is known as the progestogen-only pill because it contains no oestrogen at all. It is not quite as successful, as about one woman in five on this preparation bleeds at irregular intervals instead of having regular periods, which can be somewhat inconvenient. The failure rate is also higher, at 4 per cent. But there is still a valuable place for it where pills containing oestrogen are not advisable or not well tolerated for any reason.

From time to time the press has been full of alarms and discursions about risks associated with the Pill. Like every potent drug or medicine, there can be side-effects and sometimes these can induce a degree of risk. But it is very important to get this in perspective. No drug has ever been subjected to such prolonged, widespread and continuous assessment and tests as oestrogen. Many of the other drugs prescribed and used by doctors and patients carry far more risks, but they have not been spotlighted and emphasized in the way the tiny risks associated with oral contraception have been. Aspirin, insulin, cortisone, penicillin all save lives every day, but they also very occasionally take lives, too, and all good medicine involves accurate balance of risk and benefit.

Where the contraceptive pill is concerned the benefits are enormous. In addition to the contraceptive action, and its aesthetic appeal compared to condoms and diaphragms, a recent seven-year study of Pill-users showed considerable health bonuses quite apart from the almost 100 per cent protection against pregnancy.

Work by a team headed by Martin Vessey of Oxford University, studying 17000 British women, showed no increase in cancer of any site in Pill-users; in fact, Pill-users had fewer cancers of all types than women who used other methods.[14] This continuing study also confirmed the report of the Royal College of General Practitioners with regard to women on the Pill having markedly less benign breast disease than other women, and fewer menstrual problems.[15] The Oxford study also showed that women on the Pill were less likely to develop certain types of ovarian cysts than women using other methods of contraception, and they also had a lower rate of duodenal ulcers.

The General Practitioner survey was carried out by 1400 doctors on some 46000 women over a six-year period, and its conclusion was that the risk of serious illness associated with the Pill is minute and that women may be actually healthier when they are using the Pill. Both their study and the Oxford one confirmed the already known slightly increased risk of thrombosis, or clotting of blood in the vessels. The risk is generally set at between three and five times the norm, but it is still tiny and far less than the risk of thrombosis in actual pregnancy. Very few women among those who run into this problem actually die and only one woman in every 2000 taking the Pill will develop a blood clot. If she were pregnant, the risk would be twice as great.

The low-dosage pills have considerably reduced these risks, but even so, certain woman should not use the Pill and these include anyone who has already had a clot in a deep vein. Women who have had liver disease, severe migraine or very high blood pressure are also normally excluded, though the progestogen-only pill is sometimes used for them.

Recently there has been new evidence that the risk of thrombosis or of heart disease rises rather steeply in women over thirty-five if they also smoke or are overweight. According to the study,[16] smoking does not merely increase the danger in the older age groups but can multiply it dramatically – this effect of one drug upon the action of another is called synergistic and occurs in other cases, as with alcohol and barbiturates, for example.

If we study the figures and try to see the problem in perspective, women in their early forties who take the Pill but do *not* smoke have a mortality rate of 11 per 100000. In the same age group, for those who smoke but do *not* take the Pill, the mortality rate is 16 per 100000. So smoking is considerably more dangerous than taking the Pill. But when you put the two together and look at women who both smoke and use the Pill in the over-forty age group, then the death rate soars to 62 per 100000. Add overweight, and the risk escalates even more. A similar but much smaller effect was found in lower age groups. Even women in their twenties who smoked more than fifteen cigarettes a day and used the Pill had a higher mortality rate than similar smokers who used another contraceptive method.

So this new work really presents at least the older woman with an additional factor in her choice of contraception. If she is a smoker and unable to give it up, then she should talk over with her doctor the possibility of using other methods. But women who do not smoke, and particularly if they are not overweight either, need not really worry about the Pill if they find it, as so many do, the most acceptable and sometimes the *only* acceptable form of contraception.

Recently, very new work, both in Sweden and at the University of Wales, shows promise of further developments likely to reduce even the present small risks associated with the Pill and thrombosis. Clinical trials of the new pills in Sweden and Denmark are already under way and the development emerging from the University of Wales has already been successfully tested on animals. Production of a new pill based on this new research, however, may still take a further five years because of the stringent testing and trials, always required, and correctly so, before a new product is marketed.

Meanwhile, other common but non-dangerous side-effects of the present contraceptive pills can include such things as nausea, breast tenderness, and sometimes vomiting. But these almost always occur only in the first cycle and rapidly disappear in later usage. Some women also get occasional spotting, or breakthrough bleeding, and a few get complete absence of menstruation, but very often these can be overcome by simply changing to a different type of Pill. Pigmentation (brown freckles), increased vaginal mucus and, in just an unlucky few, some weight gain can also be experienced. Also, in a very few women, there can be migraine headaches and, in the rare susceptible individual, sometimes a rise in blood pressure.

Detailed like that it looks a formidable list, but it should be emphasized that the majority of women after the first cycle feel very well indeed on the right type of Pill. Skin, hair and energy all seem to benefit.

Depression and the Pill

There is, however, a small group (an estimated 6 per cent) of women using the Pill who run into a special form of depression rather like that experienced in PMS. Until recently there was no really successful treatment for this and when it was severe enough to be intolerable, the woman simply had to give up using the oral contraceptive. In the past it was the single biggest reason for women coming off the Pill, and it was a reason they found difficult to accept. It is one thing to give up the Pill for convincing physical or medical reasons, such as varicose veins or increased risk of thrombosis, but quite another to be forced off it because of something like depression which they felt they should be able to overcome and which somehow once again labelled them as neurotic.

Now, fortunately, research has shown that certainly in 50 per cent of such cases depression is not a neurotic reaction but has a definite physical basis. Half of all women suffering from Pill depression are found to be deficient in vitamin B6, pyridoxine.[17]

It has been known, of course, for some time that the hormones which affect the reproductive system can also profoundly affect other systems, and in these particular women the artificial hormones in the Pill blocked the action of pyridoxine, which in turn affects the tryptophan metabolism, known to affect mood and also known to be pyridoxine-dependent. This mechanism was first suggested as long ago as 1969 in papers published in the *Lancet*[18] and later work has confirmed it with many convincing trials carried out.[19]

It is now accepted that high doses of vitamin B6 can relieve Pill-related depression in at least half the women who suffer from it. The cause of depression in the other 50 per cent is still not known but work continues and no doubt an answer for them will be found in time.

While tests can be done on urine or blood samples to establish if a woman is pyridoxine-deficient, this is expensive, and most doctors today are quite simply prepared to try prescribing vitamin B6 for any woman suffering from severe depression on the Pill. A special pack is marketed for this purpose, but as it is in any case a vitamin and not a drug, pyridoxine can be bought without prescription over the counter. A point to remember, however, is that it is no use trying an ordinary replacement dose at the level at which it is normally absorbed in food. To relieve depression it has to be taken at 10 or 20 times the normal intake (that is, 50 mg or 100 mg) daily but, again, because it is a vitamin and not a drug, there are no harmful side-effects.

Starting and stopping the Pill

As we have seen, the failure rate with the Pill is almost non-existent, but this is providing it is correctly used. This means taking it regularly. Most women find this easier if they develop a routine and take it each evening. If it is forgotten, it should be taken as soon as possible the following morning, along with the usual pill for that day. This rapid 'double-up' usually prevents any pregnancy, and it should be done whether intercourse has taken place that night or not.

Another point to remember with the Pill is that it does not confer protection immediately. In the past women have been advised to start the Pill on the fifth day of their menstrual cycle and to take other contraceptive precautions for the first fourteen days. This allows time for the hormone levels to rise and suppress ovulation. Recently the Family Planning Association have come up with the bright idea of starting the Pill on the first day of the cycle (that is the first day of menstruation). With this new method the need for other temporary contraceptive measures is eliminated. The decision was taken by the FPA's medical advisory panel which includes Professor Martin Vessey, co-author of one of the recent reports quoted in this chapter; Dr Gerald Swyer of University College Hospital and a leading endocrinologist; and Dr Michael Smith, chairman and chief medical officer of the FPA. The abolition of the need for back-up contraception, together with starting the Pill four days earlier, applies also to women changing from one type of contraceptive pill to another. It should save the NHS an estimated £200000 a year if family doctors, as expected, also follow the new procedure. The saving is on the sheaths and pessaries normally supplied during the first fourteen days on the Pill. The only type of pill to which the new method is not applicable is the progestogen-only one – for it the old rules still apply.

Many women coming off the Pill to conceive a baby find ovulation returns quickly; in some instances there seems to be an increase in fertility. One study by Goldzieher found a pregnancy rate of 66 per cent in the first cycle after stopping the Pill, compared with only 35 per cent when other forms of contraception are discarded.[20] Three months after stopping the Pill, the conception rate had risen to 90 per cent.

Another study by Mears, reported that 80 per cent conceived within two months of discontinuing the Pill in London trials.[21] For this reason, because of what might be termed a bounce-back effect, the Pill is sometimes tried for infertile couples for whose problem no explanation can be found.

In contrast to this, in some women, particularly among those who have never had a child, Pill usage can cause some impairment of fertility, with women taking longer to get pregnant than those who have used other methods. In just a few cases it is necessary for women running into this temporary sterility to have sluggish ovaries prodded into action with hormone treatment; this will be discussed in Chapter 8.

Some recent evidence suggests that it might, in any case, be advisable for women over thirty-five coming off the Pill and wanting another baby to perhaps use some other form of contraception for about two months, allowing time for their bodies to settle down to normal hormone levels. This particularly applies to the thin woman over thirty-five, as the plumper woman is known to have a greater facility for manufacturing her own oestrogen. In the Jerusalem survey there appeared to be a higher incidence of abnormality in babies born to mothers over thirty-five who had conceived immediately after coming off the Pill. It was already known, of course, that babies conceived by mistake while a woman was still on the Pill could be affected. But this work is very new and a great deal more investigation is needed.

Contraception by injection

Instead of giving the hormone to suppress ovulation by mouth in the form of the Pill, it can be given by injection. In this case a progestogen-only is used, usually Depo-Provera or Norigest, but at the moment in this country both of them are only licensed for short-term use. They are particularly suitable for the short period when a couple are waiting for a vasectomy to become effective, or where a mother has had a vaccine against rubella (German measles) and needs temporary, highly effective protection until it is certain the vaccine has taken and she is not at risk from a disease which can damage the early foetus.

Longer-term clinical trials with what are termed in medical circles the 'injectables' have now been carried out, and the results are so good that the Family Planning Association is pressing for wider usage. Dr Michael Smith, their chief medical officer, believes the injections could replace the Pill for up to 100 000 women in this country.

In trials in Glasgow with Depo-Provera, the failure rate was very low indeed – only 0·25 per cent, which is the same as for the combined pill. As reported from elsewhere, however, there were some problems with irregular bleeding and weight gain, but these side-effects still only caused twelve women out of 162 to discontinue use.

The Glasgow domiciliary family planning service concluded the 'injectable' was a very valuable form of contraception not only for women unable to take the normal Pill for any reason, but also for those unable or unwilling to make regular visits to a clinic. Almost unbelievably in this day and age some women refuse to do this because of what the neighbours might think, while others are just too far away or not good at remembering to take the Pill regularly, which is essential. And then there are those whose partners will not agree to them using it.

Similar conclusions to those in Glasgow were drawn by the Charing Cross team, working with the other progestogen, Norigest. They actually found fewer problems with weight gain and bleeding on Norigest and a more rapid return to ovulation than with the Pill. This made it more suitable for women planning future pregnancies. On the debit side, however, Norigest has to be given as an injection every eight to ten weeks, while the recommended dose of Depo-Provera is only needed every twelve weeks, with a consequent saving in medical time and manpower.

There does now seem to be a strong case for the licence to be extended for more general longer usage, particularly as the method has been widely and safely employed elsewhere in the world. Depo-Provera, in particular, has been used in over 100 European and developing countries, with 19·8 million doses being injected, which adds up to five million woman-years of experience with the drug.

Despite two-thirds of users having some menstrual problems, from amenorrhoea (absence of menstruation) to the more common spotting, 80 per cent of women were happy to continue. Neither of these conditions are medically harmful but some women in the West find them psychologically unacceptable. In the developing countries the strong appeal of any medicine taken by injection probably counters these drawbacks, as the people believe it always more reliable and potent than anything just taken by mouth. Another great advantage for women in Thailand, for instance, where injectables are highly valued, is that they are ideal following childbirth: the method does not inhibit lactation in the nursing mother – in fact it may even increase the milk supply.

Even now there is nothing to stop individual doctors in Britain prescribing contraception by injection on their own responsibility and many do, particularly in the domiciliary services.

But more and more women, satisfied that their families are complete, see sterilization for themselves, or a vasectomy for their husbands, as the answer. The rather exaggerated Pill scare for the over-forties has increased the demand for both. The next chapter deals fully with the sterilization methods used and with the problem of availability.

Meanwhile, the search for the perfect contraceptive goes on and some fascinating developments are under way and, in some cases, already on trial. So let us conclude this chapter by looking at what we may hope for in the not too distant future.

Future contraceptive methods

Much current research is directed toward improving existing hormonal methods, and this has already resulted in much safer low-dosage contraceptive pills. At King's College Hospital in London they are also experimenting with adding heparin, a natural body protein which prevents blood-clotting, in the hope of eliminating the thrombosis risk at present associated with the Pill. In the first stage of the study 1000 women are being monitored and given injections of heparin on signs of clotting. It is hoped that the study may soon include a synthetic heparin, which can be taken orally as part of the Pill.

The postage-stamp pill

Some women have difficulty in swallowing tablets, however small; to overcome this and at the same time permit easier carrying and packaging, contraceptive hormones have been put into edible rice paper. Each tiny square is the size of a stamp, and can be held on or under the tongue. This has the added advantage of allowing absorption through the membranes straight into the bloodstream. It has already been approved by the government drug safety committee and is being tried out by volunteers in twenty centres in this country.

The nasal contraceptive

It sounds very way out and somehow absurd to think of taking a contraceptive by nose. Yet a nasal spray is under test at Birmingham University where the World Health Organization awarded researchers £14000 to examine the safety and effectiveness of this aerosol spray which has already been used in India. Two other centres in Oregon and New Delhi are also testing the method, which is based on traditional hormone contraception. In this country the tests are confined to Rhesus monkeys. Dr John Marston, who is in charge of the British study, told me, 'The nasal spray is believed to act directly on the hypothalamus and so we are hoping to be able to reduce the actual dose of contraceptive hormone needed.'

The contraceptive pellet

Another extension of hormone contraception is the development in Sweden of an implant which, it is claimed, will give protection for as long as six years. Known as 'chronomers', these tiny implants take the form of silicone capsules containing a supply of synthetic progesterone (D-Norgestrel) and are placed under the skin of the forearm. Only a local anaesthetic is needed and the advantages include a slow release of hormone over a longer period than any other method allows, plus easy removal if a woman decides she wishes to become pregnant. As with progestogen injections, menstrual regularity is affected.

A similar implant has also been developed at Rockefeller University in New York. There, the progestogen has been fused to a small amount of pure cholesterol, again allowing slow release of the hormone until the entire pellet is completely absorbed. Only one centimetre long, the pellet contains enough hormone to prevent conception for two to three years. Clinical trials are planned for three different versions using different progestogens.

One version, for men, includes the male hormone, testosterone, to prevent loss of libido. If the trials do prove successful, the method should be cheaper than the contraceptive pill.

Vaginal rings

New types of vaginal rings which can be inserted by the woman herself must also come into the category of research aimed at improving existing methods. The present IUDs, of course, have to be put in and taken out by a doctor.

The World Health Organization has announced research

into a ring which releases contraceptive hormones throughout a three-month lifespan and is then renewed by the user. In both the US and Belgium, a silicone vaginal ring, impregnated with progesterone, is being tested; it can be fitted round the cervix by the woman herself, left for three weeks, and then taken out to allow one week of withdrawal bleed before a new ring is inserted.

The egg-timer

This is what I suppose might be termed the 'fun' name applied to various devices being developed to try and pinpoint onset of ovulation. Again it is a question of improving on an existing system. Doctors in some forty-six countries, with the ardent backing of the Catholic Church, are working to bring a degree of accuracy into what was really only a very hit-or-miss system.

In Dublin doctors claim to have produced a magic box which can detect electric charges in a woman's body when she ovulates. Rather more hopefully in Glasgow, Professor Ian Donald is on the track of a method which detects changes in the pelvis when the egg ripens. 'Eventually it could take the form of a dip-stick,' he explains, 'which when applied to the vagina would change colour to show when a woman is fertile.'

Professor Donald's idea is not so way-out as it might seem for, in America, the Harvard Medical School have already come up with a simple form of 'viscometer'. They claim this instrument is able to measure the fluidity of the cervical mucus, which is known to change some twelve to eighteen hours *before* ovulation. Although it was devised originally to help women who wanted to conceive (because it would indicate ovulation so well in advance), it would obviously have even greater potential as an inexpensive and apparently easy-to-understand method of determining the 'safe' period. Tests to determine its accuracy are currently taking place.

These would appear to be proving acceptable, as a machine rather grandly termed an Ovutime Fertility Detection System is already being used in fertility clinics in America, where it is claimed the mucus sample is obtained in seconds and the results are available instantly. It is hardly convenient to have to go to a clinic every time you want to check your ovulation day, but work is now going on with a home pocket-version no bigger than a packet of cigarettes. If this does prove accurate it could be available in the UK around 1979, at the cost of around £14. In the long term it could be argued that is cheaper than the Pill, providing it is also going to be equally effective.

This Ovutime method would still demand the degree of discipline required to refrain from intercourse at the specified times if conception was to be avoided. This clearly makes it unsuitable for the young, who really do not want to have to consult a time-machine or egg-timer before deciding if they can make love, and anyway they are not usually worried about the Pill. But it could be useful for the older, married woman wanting to plan her family.

Another similar method known as the Muthermic Method relies on the same principle but insists that use of a thermometer combined with a little instruction can enable women to determine the condition of the mucus and accurately predict ovulation. I have to admit my own reservations after seeing so many disasters through reliance on the so-called natural or rhythm methods, but I suppose one should keep on open mind and see what sort of failure and success rates emerge.

The sponge contraceptive

Although this has to be placed in a second category of really new methods, and the University of Arizona where it is being tested hails it as a 'future advance', it actually sounds at first more like reversion to an age-old method. In Roman times sponges were sometimes soaked in vinegar in the hope that they would act as a contraceptive by blocking the entry to the uterus. The new method, however, does at least use a new type of soft non-irritating sponge, which needs to be removed only during menstruation and can be washed and reinserted.

Vaccination against pregnancy

This falls into the category of contraception based on a truly new principle.

The Medical Research Council's unit in Edinburgh has already tested one form but so far only with monkeys. It immunizes against a substance produced in the brain which stimulates production of the reproductive hormones. The substance, known as luteinizing hormone-releasing factor, is produced in the hypothalamus part of the brain, passes in the bloodstream to the pituitary gland and there stimulates release of the vital luteinizing hormone (LH) and follicle-stimulating hormone (FSH) which, as described earlier (see pages 22–24), control the production of oestrogen and progesterone in women.

But the same substance also controls development of sperm in the male and production of the male hormone, testosterone. A synthetic preparation of the hormone has been found (together with another ingredient that intensifies the effect) to produce antibodies which prevent the whole chain-reaction starting up. So this new work, now being taken up in many countries, offers promise of a male contraceptive as well as a female one, both likely to be long-lasting, inexpensive and reversible. But the work is in its early stages and, as always, long periods of clinical trials with human volunteers must lie ahead before effectiveness and safety can be guaranteed for general use.

In Belgium related research revolves round a new hormone isolated from the male testes, called inhibin, which has also been shown to suppress the FSH produced by the pituitary to stimulate sperm production. This again holds out hope for the development of a male contraceptive, but also for helping to cure some forms of male infertility, which may be associated with raised inhibin levels.

Harvard Medical School, obviously very active in contraceptive research, also report work testing an anti-sperm-production compound, known as indazol carboxylic acid. Again, so far it has only been proved in monkeys, where a daily dose has been shown to arrest sperm production and infertility, maintained afterwards by a once-a-week dose.

The 'anti-baby' vaccine, as it has been called in the popular press, has been hailed as the ultimate in contraception. It has been forecast that by the end of the century teenagers could be vaccinated so that they deliberately opt out of reproduction until they are able and ready to make the decision to start a family.

Beside the methods already described and under test, some doctors believe it may be possible to produce drugs that will make a girl immune to male sperm. Just a few women do show allergic reaction to sperm. One girl was reported breaking out in a rash, spasms and fits of sneezing. Another developed a rash and asthma with lips, eyelids, tongue and throat swollen and violent pains in the pelvis.

It is probably wise to warn that all this is very speculative, but it is also known that in just a few cases infertility can be caused by the husband developing antibodies to his own sperm. Antibodies are described in more detail in Chapter 8, but they are part of the immune mechanism and so it is possible that eventually women or men could be in some way immunized, men against their own sperm and women against tissues produced in pregnancy such as placenta. But even the most optimistic estimate for this sort of radical advance is another twenty years.

The morning-after pill

This is another colourful lay press term for what is medically known as a post-coital pill, used simply after each session of intercourse.

Work on this has tended to centre round a substance called prostaglandin. But recently a new approach, using a synthetic version of the second female hormone, offers considerable hope. We have already referred to these progestogens; one called D-Norgestrel, taken within three hours of intercourse, has yielded a low pregnancy rate of only 1·69 per cent, which compares more than favourably with pre-coital continuous methods such as the Pill. The only snag is that three hours, because used after that time the failure rate rises steeply.

In cases of rape, providing a woman goes at once to a doctor, effective action with high doses of oestrogen can be taken. A synthetic potent oestrogen called ethinyloestradiol is most often used – 5 mg a day for five days, and within twenty-four to thirty-six hours at the latest. Professor Haspells, the Royal Gynaecologist of Holland, whom I met at a Menopause Symposium at which I was speaking in Athens, described his own study involving 2000 women. The only failures that occurred were in women on doses of oestrogen lower than 5 mg and he now considers this the standard effective minimum.

Both prostaglandin and high-dose oestrogen can produce side-effects such as nausea, vomiting and sometimes breast tenderness and irregular bleeding. While the high dose of oestrogen needed can be used with confidence on a single occasion, and most certainly to counter something like pregnancy resulting from rape, it might present a health hazard if used routinely, and should certainly never be looked upon as an easy or regular back-up to replace normal contraception.

An even better method of post-coital protection may lie in work going on with a copper-containing IUD. It has been recognized that these devices work by preventing implantation of the fertilized egg and as this may take up to six days after ovulation, it may be possible to prevent by insertion of an IUD soon after intercourse. Early reports are very encouraging and the fact that there are few adverse side-effects could make it more acceptable than the present methods. In addition, of course, the IUD would then be in place to provide further continuing protection.

The search for the male contraceptive

It has often seemed a little unfair that women seem to be the ones who not only have to accept the risks and discomfort of pregnancy and childbirth, but also the risks and responsibility of preventing it.

Biologists argued that it was technically easier to influence the mechanism of the female, which produces usually just one single egg a month, than to try and interfere with the continuous production of sperm. There has proved to be truth in this, but undoubtedly there have also been some psychological barriers in men's dislike of accepting personal responsibility for contraception, and in their deep-seated and totally mistaken belief that fertility and potency are somehow connected.

In the 1950s there was considerable excitement about a male contraceptive pill being tried out which seemed to inhibit sperm production. Unfortunately it proved to be incompatible with alcohol so, needless to say, it was ruled out.

The second problem encountered is that most drugs, including oestrogens and progestogens, which inhibit the production of FSH and LH and so break the chain-reaction leading to sperm production, also prevent or reduce production of testosterone, the male hormone related to sex drive. Obviously if libido is reduced the method will yet again prove unacceptable.

Recent work, however, is based on combining such drugs with replacement testosterone to avoid a fall in libido. Testosterone itself strangely enough suppresses FSH and LH but to do so requires large doses and this involves questions of long-term safety. Slow-release pellets of testosterone under the skin may provide a safer answer. Meanwhile in Australia, a combination of synthetic methyltestosterone and an oestrogen which could be taken by mouth suppressed sperm production in four out of five volunteers. But again two of them complained of some decrease in libido, although it was not certain if this was directly due to the drug or to a psychological reaction because the user expected it.

Very recently another combination of testosterone and a weak male hormone derivative called Danazol has been shown to reduce sperm production in eleven out of thirteen men without any effect on libido.

And so the work goes on, but the best prospect for a male Pill seems to lie in the development of combinations which will prevent the chain-reaction ever starting by preventing the production of the initial luteinizing-hormone-releasing factor. What is also needed, however, is a simple fertility test for men, a method which would make it possible to decide if the sperm count had been reduced sufficiently to ensure conception could not take place, or if the sperm present had been 'incapacitated' sufficiently to prevent them being able to penetrate the egg. This relates to a second possible method of contraception for men which, rather than suppressing sperm production and interfering with testosterone and libido, might rely instead on preventing the sperm maturing and becoming 'capacitated', to use the medical phrase.

If sperm could be kept immature and 'incapacitated', they would not be active enough to achieve fertilization. One drug has already been found to work in this way, but adverse side-effects in trials with monkeys has so far prevented it from being used for human trials.

Any new drugs developed have to be tested on many thousands of men over long periods to ensure safety and a return to fertility when desired. So there can be no swift and sure solution to the problems of contraception within the near future, at least in terms of a male contraceptive. But in more general terms the prospect is bright and John Newton, consultant gynaecologist at King's College Hospital, London, one of Britain's leading birth control experts, told me:

I believe we are on the verge of a tremendous breakthrough with new and safer contraceptive methods, which will not interfere with a woman's own hormone levels. At King's College we are testing under licence means of delivering effective spermicidal substances in such concentrations that there should be no chance of sperm surviving or penetrating. One method uses a vaginal ring which the woman puts in herself, but the other involves the doctor placing a specially shaped device containing the spermicide actually in the narrow cervical canal. So far the methods appear successful and safe and if all continues to go well should be available within around five years.

So the future is bright, but meanwhile it is time to consider sterilization which, once their family is complete, more and more couples see as the best available method of contraception.

6. Sterilization

Perhaps because sterilization and abortion both involve surgical techniques and are widely used throughout the world as means of fertility control, they are sometimes linked in people's minds.

In fact, sterilization is a purely contraceptive measure, based on the principle of closing off the tubes to prevent passage of the egg in the female or sperm in the male. In contrast, abortion involves actual destruction of the already fertilized egg or embryo, which, whatever your moral viewpoint, puts it into an entirely different ethical category.

In our own society there is one strong link between them. At the moment in Great Britain both are perfectly legal, subject to certain conditions, but there remain in both cases wild discrepancy and injustice in their availability. This is invariably rooted in the attitudes and priorities of gynaecologists and/or in the funding problems and priorities of the Health Authorities in different areas.

So in the next two chapters we shall be dealing not only with the medical aspects of the very different surgical procedures involved, but also with the very similar problems encountered in getting them done, and the way in which our system works, or too often fails to work, with provision being either too little or too late.

In considering sterilization, the first thing most people ask is if the operation will affect sex hormone levels or sexual feeling. The answer, for both the man having a vasectomy or the woman undergoing any form of female sterilization, is a firm and reassuring 'No'. Women continue to have the same sex hormone levels, to ovulate and to menstruate. The idea that periods are sometimes heavier after the female operation is not borne out by the studies so far done. The eggs that are ripened and released each month, but whose passage down the fallopian tubes is blocked, are simply reabsorbed, perfectly naturally, by the body, as are thousands of other unused eggs in the course of a lifetime, with or without sterilization.

After a male vasectomy, too, there are no changes in hormone levels and no loss of sex drive, except occasionally when a man is worried that there will be.

The most important thing is for both partners to understand that sterilization should be considered a permanent operation. With existing techniques it is never possible to guarantee reversal, so both should be agreed on the step to be taken and satisfied they will not want more children.

At the moment a great deal of work is going on with female sterilization, using a laparoscope technique and employing rubber rings and clips to seal off the tubes in the hope that these methods may allow for easier reversal, but it is too early yet to know how successful this will be. Many believe that the clip method holds out good hope.

However for the moment the operation for either men or women is supposed to be free and available only on the understanding that it is considered permanent. Subject to proper counselling about this and careful consideration by the couple, the Department of Health and Social Security positively encourage this permanent form of birth control, on both medical and on social grounds, to any couple who simply feel they have all the children they want and can cope with. The DHSS do advise that both partners consent, but in practice it is interesting that while consent is almost always sought from the husband when a woman applies for sterilization, it is by no means always sought from the wife when a man applies for vasectomy.

Officially encouraged in this way, and with the recent Pill scare in relation to older women adding further impetus, there is strong pressure for sterilization. One Family Planning doctor told me:

Women over 40 at our clinic don't want to come off the Pill, but unfortunately they don't want to give up smoking either, and most of them find they can't. So if they smoke heavily, some try switching to a diaphragm or an IUD, but even more tend to apply for sterilization or their husbands for vasectomy.

Female sterilization

The initial operation to close the fallopian tubes is done either by cutting and tying them, or by destroying part of them by cauterization (heat). At one time this usually involved opening the abdomen, but usually now it can be done far more simply with the invaluable laparoscope. This consists of a narrow tube, fitted with a viewing lens, down which the surgeon can actually look into the body. He can also use part of the tube to pass down delicate instruments and use them to perform some forms of surgery. With this method only a small incision is needed and it considerably cuts down the stay in hospital.

At St Mary's Hospital in London many sterilizations using a laparoscope are actually done under local anaesthetic; and this is very common in America. But even where a general anaesthetic is used many hospitals now use laparoscope techniques and treat the minor operation as a day case. In Aberdeen, which is one of the places where this is done and where so much good medicine for women has been pioneered, women come in at 8 a.m., after fasting since midnight. The patient can always stay the night if she prefers, but is normally free to go home at 5 p.m., with just a supply of paracetamol tablets, which is all that is usually needed to relieve any pain.

A follow-up study at Aberdeen has shown the method to be so free of complications that family doctors reported only 7 per cent of patients with even minor post-operative problems. None needed to be referred back to hospital, and 90 per cent of the patients were back to normal on the fourth day.

The chances of reversal

The method used for the initial sterilization very much affects the chances of reversal, but in any case it is always a far bigger and more difficult operation. Mr Robert Beard, one of our leading gynaecologists, attached to the Royal Sussex Hospital in Brighton, told me:

Attempted reversal for women requires a bigger incision than for the original sterilization. It requires also a longer anaesthetic, more days in hospital and a longer convalescence.

If only a small part of the centre of the tube has been removed or destroyed, then it's relatively simple to join it together again, with pregnancy resulting in 50 to 60 per cent of cases. But if the tube has been destroyed at its point of entry to the womb, then it's a much bigger operation with far less chance of success. Also if a baby is subsequently conceived, it will need to be delivered by Caesarean section. [This, of course, means through the abdomen by another surgical operation.]

Mr Beard went on to outline the most difficult problem of all. 'That is when the outer end of the tube has been removed in the original sterilization,' he explained. 'Then a new opening must be fashioned and it's seldom successful with at most a 10 per cent chance of pregnancy. Also it leads to more chance of ectopic or tubal pregnancy at the site of the new junction, and this always means a termination.'

As a final warning he added, 'There's no way of knowing what situation applies until the abdomen is opened at the time of trying for reversal, or by doing a laparoscopic examination first.'

All this makes it very clear how important proper counselling and careful consideration must always be. But there are plenty of cases where this has been done and where a woman and her husband both agree on sterilization, her own family doctor puts her name forward and still she finds herself refused. From my own researches I have discovered that if the cash runs out in any particular area, the sterilizations have to stop. What is more, if the top gynaecologist puts sterilization low on his list of priorities, they may not even start.

This can fall hard on the woman for whom normal methods of contraception are either unacceptable or more often medically unsuitable. One women I met, Dorothy Mason, perfectly illustrates this point. At only thirty-two she found herself pregnant for the eighth time. She already had five living children, aged fifteen, fourteen, eleven, nine and seven. Of these the fourteen-year-old had fits and the seven-year-old was mentally handicapped. On top of this Dorothy looked after her mother who was epileptic and her unemployed husband who had had a heart attack. She told me, 'We tried all the usual birth control methods but always came unstuck until we tried the Pill. That worked fine but the doctor had to take me off because of thrombosis risk.'

Dorothy had already had two NHS abortions, each time requesting sterilization to be performed afterwards, when it is a relatively simple additional procedure. *Each time, incredibly, she was refused.* 'In desperation the third time we scraped together some money,' she told me, 'and I had both done together under the British Pregnancy Advisory Service. Even so we had to have a partial loan, which we're still struggling to pay back. I don't understand the situation, because if free NHS sterilization isn't meant for people like me, then who is it meant for?'

It's a good question and one the British Pregnancy Advisory Service also asks hundreds of times a week, as women apply to them after being refused by the NHS or only promised a place on hopelessly long waiting lists.

BPAS is a registered charity which seeks to plug the often appalling gaps in NHS provision both of sterilization and abortion. From their headquarters at Austry Manor, Wootten Wawen, Solihull, West Midlands B95 6DA, it is possible to get details of the network of clinics and services they run across the country. By employing doctors on a sessional basis, BPAS keep costs to a minimum, but even so, for Dorothy the cost of the two surgical procedures and two nights in a BPAS clinic, plus nursing and counselling care, was £72·50 – a lot of money to find for a service not only supposed to be free, but one which the Department of Health and Social Security has so deliberately set out to advertise and promote.

I came across all too many similar cases during my research in 1977, and it's clear that the borderline between social and medical sterilizations is very blurred.

Mary, another thirty-two-year-old mother I talked to, had already lost one baby before going on to achieve the family of three which was all she and her husband felt they could cope with. 'After the fourth birth I used the Pill,' she explained, 'but unfortunately I put on two stones in weight and this plus varicose veins meant my doctor insisted I should come off.'

Like Dorothy, when she became pregnant Mary was granted an NHS abortion but refused a sterilization. As her husband would not have a vasectomy she had a coil inserted. 'This had to be removed,' she told me, 'because it perforated the womb. The next time I got pregnant, to be fair, they did promise me another NHS abortion and this time a sterilization. But the waiting time was going to be so long that I would have been over fourteen weeks pregnant before it was done and I didn't fancy that. So instead we borrowed the money and paid under BPAS.'

In Mary's case the gynaecologist obviously considered that her sterilizations were non-urgent and came under the 'social' category; or it could be that he also objected to doing this particular operation on a relatively young woman. At any rate it came low on his list of priorities. One gynaecologist explained his own attitude to me quite bluntly. 'Once sterilizations were encouraged,' he argued, 'they were bound to compete with other procedures which I consider more urgent. The job of a gynaecologist in my view is to treat the ill and the sick, not to have time taken up with what must be termed "social medicine".'

Even on medical grounds, however, I found no guarantee of free sterilization in this man's area. At the same hospital, a Jamaican woman with five children told me that, according to the doctor she had just seen, her only hope was to have the operation done privately, when there would be no waiting involved.

Leaving out the cost in terms of anxiety and stress, which cannot ever be estimated, it is still a crazy situation in strict economic terms. Women refused sterilization go on to be a far greater charge on the NHS, with unwanted pregnancies, costly abortions or the equally costly alternative of many years of free contraception – free to them, but expensive for the NHS and the tax-payer who funds it.

Fortunately there are other gynaecologists who recognize this, and the woman's and her husband's rights in the matter. Mr Joe Jordan, consultant gynaecologist at Birmingham Maternity Hospital and Birmingham Women's Hospital, has said:

We should not reject demands for sterilizations from men or women because in our opinion they are too young or have too few children. They should be given proper counselling, with the probability that the operation is irreversible fully explained, but after they have given consideration to all this, the aim of the service must be to allow people to make their own decision, and to have the number of children *they* want at the time *they* want them.

A great deal of the muddle and lack of finance stems from Barbara Castle's insistence in 1975 that all hospital doctors carrying out family planning should receive special payment. They had not asked for this and many vociferously opposed it, but Mrs Castle argued that the work fell outside their contracts and that it would bring them into line with the GPs, who were already being paid extra for this work.

It is difficult to defend one medical service being separated out for special payment in this way. There seems little reason to discriminate between tying off fallopian tubes and dealing with varicose veins.

Perhaps at the time free family planning was seen as an important vote-catcher with the general public, and extra pay as a soothing syrup to bring down the temperature of the hospital doctors, already in a fevered state over finance and conditions of work.

Whatever the motives, the outcome unfortunately was the same, with tax-payers' money misspent, patients failing to benefit, and even doctors given reason for discontent, as the money is just not available to fund the service properly, and making availability dependent on the priority it is given by each individual Area Health Authority. Apart from making more money available, there are two practical measures which could be taken and for which women should be pressing. One is the fullest use of laparoscope techniques and more day-care provision, and the other is greater availability of vasectomies and better education of men so that they will use this service, which is not only easier and safer than female sterilization but much cheaper.

Vasectomy

Vasectomy is not only simpler and cheaper as already stated, but is also the most effective of all means of contraception yet known, with the lowest failure rate of only 0·1 per cent, or one in a thousand.

The operation involves only a quick out-patient procedure, under local anaesthetic with little discomfort. The tube through which the sperm reaches the semen (sex fluid) lies in a pouch of skin (scrotum). A tiny incision is made in this pouch, the tube (vas deferens) gently pulled out and snipped through, then replaced and the small wound covered with sticking plaster. The procedure takes about fifteen minutes and, after a short rest, the man can walk away.

Although couples are warned that the operation is never to be considered reversible even for the man, in fact 45 per cent of male tubes can be successfully rejoined and result in renewed fertility. It's important for couples also to be warned that a vasectomy is not immediately effective, as millions of sperm will already be in the semen, and these have to be used up through ejaculation before possible pregnancy from intercourse can be ruled out. Tests are usually carried out over a period of three to four months, until the doctor is satisfied the semen is sperm-free. During that time other means of contraception must be used.

With proper counselling before any decision is taken, few men ever regret vasectomy, but it is important that they should not be pressured into it and should make up their own minds, as otherwise there can sometimes be adverse psychological reactions.

It is such a simple solution to the contraceptive problem for a couple whose family is complete that it is surprising how few men have been prepared in the past to have this minor surgery done. The trouble has almost certainly been because of lingering myths confusing vasectomy with castration, and some men imagining they would develop falsetto voices, breasts and fat buttocks like a eunuch. In fact the testicles are not even touched, let alone removed and, as already stated, the male hormone levels remain the same. *Most important of all, virility is unimpaired.* In fact a vasectomy can often have exactly the opposite effect, perhaps through the better relationship and response that becomes possible when a woman is relieved of all fear of pregnancy or of the Pill.

Better information in schools on this subject, as part of better general contraceptive education, might do a lot towards eliminating these old unjustified fears before they get a grip on yet another generation.

Meanwhile, happily, more and more men are coming forward for vasectomies, and it has become vital to increase the availability of the service to meet the demand. Vasectomies actually save the NHS money both on surgeons' fees (and on the anaesthetists' fees which are involved in female sterilization) and in nursing and in hospital stay, neither of which are required with vasectomy.

In 1977 I found only thirty-nine of the Area Health Authorities (less than half) were then fulfilling their obligation to provide a free vasectomy service, despite funds allocated by the DHSS to try to get the scheme off the ground. Since then, however, efforts have been made to bring about a fairer distribution of finance and facilities to help the medically deprived areas.

Individual women and women's movements may still need to exert pressure, however, in areas where gynaecologists' attitudes are holding back proper provision of either vasectomies, sterilizations or abortions

7. Abortion

People who, like myself, have over the years campaigned for more liberal abortion laws and welcomed David Steel's Bill in 1967 as bringing the law into the twentieth century, are sometimes accused of being in *favour* of abortion.

The truth is no one could ever be in favour of abortion, except in those cases where it has to be undertaken for strictly medical reasons, to save a mother's life or prevent a very badly damaged baby being brought into the world.

In almost every other instance abortion is a confession of failure – a failure of education, a failure of contraception, a failure of the system.

In an ideal world with an ideal society composed of ideal people, abortion would never be necessary except in the special circumstances just mentioned. But we have to deal with the world and with society realistically, and with individuals as they are and as they behave, not how we would like them to behave.

So, with this in mind, abortion can often be seen as the lesser of evils, and always a lesser evil than the birth of an unwanted child into a crowded world, where someday unless we get things right, even wanted children may have to be limited to solve an overall population problem.

Of course there should always be proper counselling and discussion; of course every sort of help and support should always be offered, so that no woman who really wants to keep her child should ever feel pressured into a termination. And although I believe sterilizations should be given when they are wanted at the time of abortion, no woman should ever be granted an abortion *only* if she agrees to a sterilization. That sometimes happens at the moment with a woman already under stress asked to make such a vital long-term decision.

But providing the options are explained and the help available outlined, if a woman still decides she wants a termination, then I believe it is her right to have one, but as *early* in her pregnancy as it can be done.

Any such termination should be accompanied by sterilization if it is really wanted and the matter has been fully considered with no pressure applied. If sterilization is not wanted then good contraceptive advice to avoid further abortions should be obligatory, and this is part of the policy under BPAS regulations and is also supposed to be done under NHS.

The law on abortion

It might be helpful to set out as simply as possible the main provisions of the 1967 Abortion Act. Under this, termination of pregnancy is legally permitted up to the twenty-eighth week for any one of the following reasons:

If your life is at greater risk by continuing with the pregnancy than by terminating it.

If your physical or mental health is more likely to be injured by continuing with the pregnancy than by terminating.

If the physical or mental health of any existing children you have is more likely to be injured by your continuing pregnancy than by terminating it.

If there is a reasonable chance that the baby may be abnormal or deformed.

The law requires that you are seen by two doctors and that both agree that termination is justified. Under the present system one of these doctors may or may not be your own GP, but the other is usually likely to be the clinic doctor or hospital gynaecologist who will carry out the operation, *if* he interprets the law in favour of termination. The decision is likely to depend on the way one or both doctors choose to interpret the law, and that will depend on their attitude to abortion generally and your situation particularly. If you are under sixteen, one of your parents must sign a consent form to the operation.

The vital early pregnancy test

If termination can be done early it is simple and very safe.

Before the tenth week of pregnancy is safest of all, but right up to the first twelve weeks the mortality rate is only 1·7 per 100 000 operations, far lower than in pregnancy. In comparison, having your tonsils out is twice as dangerous as early abortion, and hysterectomy (removal of the womb) is 120 times as dangerous. But the relative risk of termination after that goes up after the tenth week and at the eighteenth week it is forty-five times more dangerous. So the later the abortion the more dangerous, and the bigger the operation the more disagreeable for all concerned.

All this makes it very important to have a pregnancy test done early, particularly if you are thinking of asking for termination. An accurate positive result can be obtained from a specimen of urine, taken first thing on waking, as early as ten to fourteen days after a period is overdue (that is six weeks after the first day of your last period, if you have a twenty-eight-day cycle). Two or three tablespoons of urine in a clean bottle are enough, and it should be labelled with your full name, date of collection of the specimen, and date of the first day of your last menstrual period.

It is best to seek the advice of your own doctor, but if for any reason you do not want to do this, then a confidential pregnancy test can be arranged for you through your local Family Planning Clinic, Brook Clinic or BPAS. Citizens Advice Bureaux and local Welfare Officers may also be able to steer you in the right direction for help.

While a positive test indicates pregnancy even at this early stage, it should be noted that at only fourteen days a negative test may not invariably be correct, and to be sure it should be repeated again two weeks later. If the test is again negative but you miss a second period, it is *essential* to have it done yet again.

But the whole point of early testing is that if pregnancy is confirmed and you decide to have a termination, you can get it arranged in good time. Remember if you are in a difficult area, the delays involved and the shopping around you may have to do will hold things up.

These days one sees 'do-it-yourself pregnancy test' kits advertised quite widely, and it is not difficult to imagine circumstances in which this must seem a tempting solution particularly for the shy girl who may feel it will avoid embarrass-ment. The only trouble is that if there is a margin of error, as we have already seen, in *professional* testing, then there is even more chance of a mistake in any 'do-it-yourself' system. Cer-tainly in the early stages no doctor is prepared to rely simply on one chemical test and nor can you. The self-testing methods can give both false negatives which may lull you into a false sense of security, if you have been hoping you are not pregnant, and false positives which in the same circumstances may involve unnecessary worry. It is best they should only be considered as preliminary checks, particularly where a positive result comes up.

What does abortion involve?

Termination any time within the first three months usually involves only one night in a hospital or clinic. In some areas out-patient abortions are available at this early stage. The methods used are either what is called vacuum suction or vacuum aspiration, which is really much as it sounds, with the unwanted content of the uterus being sucked out through a tube; alternatively a D and C, or dilation and curettage, is given, involving gently dilating or stretching the neck of the womb and scraping the contents out. The vacuum method is sometimes done with a local anaesthetic.

As a matter of interest and perhaps to reassure the very sensitive, even a doctor cannot distinguish on later examination between someone who has had a deliberate termination by suction abortion and a normal miscarriage.

From the fourth month of pregnancy onwards these simple techniques are no longer possible. One of the two methods most commonly used for later terminations is a sort of mini-Caesarean section in which the abdomen is opened, and recovery from this obviously takes longer with a stay of about six days in hospital. The other, and preferable method is a medically induced termination which brings on a form of labour usually lasting between twelve and thirty-six hours. The pregnancy over, it is usually possible to leave hospital about twenty-four hours later with this method.

There are a number of minor side-effects that may occur no

matter which method is used. A woman who is too energetic during the forty-eight hours following the operation may find she gets heavy bleeding, in which case bed rest is necessary.

Blood loss following an abortion varies a great deal from patient to patient. It may finish after a few days like a period, or it may dribble on for two or three weeks. Some women experience intermittent cramp-like pains for a few days afterwards, especially if a number of small blood clots are being passed. Undue or sudden pain or excessive bleeding, rise in temperature, or increased feeling of illness, should always be reported. These symptoms rarely occur and can be treated safely, providing you inform a doctor straight away.

As the neck of the womb will remain open for a while after most types of operation for termination, there is a slight risk of infection occurring. To reduce this risk tampons or other internal protection should not be used and you should avoid sitting or lying in a bath for a week after the operation. Intercourse should be avoided for at least two weeks, longer if possible.

In my experience, talking to many women following abortion, I have to say that their main reaction was one of relief and gratitude. But other researchers and doctors occasionally report an emotional backlash and even a guilt complex in women. This seems to be more likely with late abortion, and could perhaps be aggravated by the onset of lactation which some women may find occurring, so it is best to realize that this can happen with a termination from the fourth month onwards.

In general I feel sure that much of the backlash and guilt which has been experienced in the past has been due to the harrowing and guilt-inducing attitudes encountered. The dangers and very real risks of abortion, together with nervous reactions, were the product of the old bad laws which forced women to bad and dangerous back-street abortions. Today legal abortion carries neither risks nor reaction except in rare cases, and the most recent study of post-abortion psychosis reported in 1977 in the *British Medical Journal* confirmed an incidence of only 0·3 per 1000 for legal abortions, against an incidence of 1·7 per 1000 deliveries for post-natal psychosis. Dr Colin Brewer, who had the help of twenty-one psychiatrists in carrying out this study, concluded greater emotional turmoil can be caused by childbirth and child-rearing, whether welcome or not, and that this may be linked to the more profound hormonal and other physiological changes involved.[22]

So this first and very recent scientific study bears out the contention that it was the operation of the law rather than the operation of the skilled doctors which produced problems. David Steel's Bill, if allowed to work as it was intended, was designed to sweep away privilege. Unfortunately, as we have already seen with the far less controversial issue of sterilization, there can still be gross injustice and a veritable obstacle race to be run in some areas, set up by medical attitudes which determine how the law is interpreted.

With abortion, the examples of local discrimination can be even more striking. Ten years after the new Abortion Law, only 50 per cent of terminations are yet being done under the NHS. If these were spread evenly across the country, there might be some argument that it at least represented social justice in the form of equal opportunity or lack of it. But there are vast variations in NHS provision. In Wolverhampton for example, only 7 per cent of patients can get an NHS abortion, in Birmingham only 10 per cent and in Coventry only 16 per cent. Yet in Bristol, the figure rises to 65 per cent, in Newcastle and Aberdeen 96 per cent and in Scotland as a whole 88 per cent.

The contrast between Newcastle and Birmingham is particularly interesting, because although the chance of actually getting an abortion in the two cities is roughly equal, this is entirely thanks to a very efficient branch of BPAS in Birmingham, where nine out of ten women have to buy their treatment privately. In Newcastle nine out of ten can obtain abortion free under NHS.

Obviously no consultant with religious or genuine moral objections to abortion should ever be forced to do them, but neither should he or she be able to impose values or prejudices to influence provision over an entire area. This is certainly happening at the moment, particularly with consultants holding influential posts attached to teaching hospitals.

The DHSS have tried to overcome the problem in two ways. First by reminding Area Health Authorities of their obligations to provide a full service, and secondly by suggesting where patients might suffer if a post being offered were filled by yet

D

another anti-abortion doctor, then the job description must clearly state commitment to perform such operations. This worked well in 1976, with the procedure only proving necessary for fourteen out of 193 vacancies. All the same, the Select Committee on Abortion recommended the system be dropped in case it affected career prospects for any particular doctor. This seems extraordinary when you consider that the anti-abortion views of just one doctor can affect the lives and rights of thousands of women.

It is possible that the good work being done by the charitable pregnancy advisory services in filling the gaps left by the NHS allow feet to be dragged. The Select Committee's other recommendation to solve the problem of provision, by establishing separate abortion units in particular hospitals, has not been followed up in many areas. Nor has the obvious solution of day-care services, already proving economic, safe and efficient both for early abortion and for sterilization.

It's puzzling, not only that these obvious solutions proceed so slowly, but that efforts go on to try to limit existing provision, in the face of the fact that two in five doctors already admit to difficulty in referring patients for abortion and, three-quarters of them confirmed approval of the present law.

To reinforce this, in 1977 a letter was sent to Social Services Minister, David Ennals, on behalf of 2000 doctors including more than 50 per cent of Britain's professors of obstetrics, asking for any details of the working of the present Act, which would possibly justify attempts such as Mr Benyon's Bill to restrict the law. The BMA conference in Glasgow during the same year made a strong recommendation for the present law to be retained, and since then a group of doctors calling themselves 'Doctors for a Woman's Choice in Abortion' have set out to produce a report with the object of getting unfair regional variations in provision put right.

The last National Opinion Poll in 1976 showed 55 per cent of the general public approved abortion on request; meanwhile, under the present law, the peak abortion level of 1973 has continued to drop, with 1976 showing a figure of 9 per cent lower than 1975 and representing one of the lowest rates in Europe. Twenty-nine countries now have liberal abortion laws, and it would be entirely against the trend of both public and medical opinion to make our own legislation more restrictive. As Dr Malcolm Potts, director of the International Fertility Research Programme, points out:

With the added delays amending legislation would inevitably produce, the losers would be those least able to cope, the very young and couples least blessed in education. They deserve sympathy and help, not the deliberate creation of expensive, slow acting, unnecessarily dangerous services. The only ones to gain would be the very group of doctors whose activities such legislation purports to control.

Certainly at present the initial commercial abuses have been eliminated; the touting for customers, high charges and poor conditions of some private clinics have been done away with. Clinics now have to meet proper medical standards before being given a licence and their numbers are strictly limited.

Before the present Act, abortion abuses were on a far wider scale and if anyone wants an object lesson on the evils of restrictive abortion, the latest figures from South America are a horrific example. Where legal and safe abortion is not offered, women resort to illegal and unsafe abortion. The Bolivian Ministry of Public Health estimates that the treatment of complications from illegal abortions accounts for more than 60 per cent of all their costs in caring for patients. The largest maternity hospital in Bogotà, Colombia, devotes half its beds to similar cases and a recent study showed abortion as the major cause of death among women between fifteen and thirty-five. In Venezuela abortion accounts for 70 per cent of the high maternal death rate. Throughout the world, despite the breakthrough in abortion reform in some countries, 150000 women are still estimated to die from illegal abortion each year – sacrificed to Catholic conscience and unrealistic unworkable laws. The terrible irony is that, denied contraception, it is Catholic women who pour into this country for abortion – from Spain, Italy, Portugal and Ireland. The total number of non-resident women who had abortions in England and Wales during the first quarter of this year was 8182, the highest number from any country coming from Spain. But the numbers from Ireland are still rising – 1406 in 1974, 1562 in 1975 and 1802 in 1976. In the first three months alone of 1977, 501 Irish women came here for termination according to statistics released by the Office of Population Censuses and Surveys.

This subject has commanded a lot of space in my book because women need to be on guard against the attempts which will undoubtedly go on to take away the hard-won right to legal abortion under the conditions which have been democratically approved. Minority anti-abortionists are able to exert overt pressure through the powerful communication network offered by the Catholic Church.

Women have no such organization at their command, but they do have the support of the majority of doctors who want to see the present Bill retained. And they also have the support of men like Professor Peter Huntingford of the London Hospital, Mr Peter Diggory at Kingston and Mr John McGarry at Barnstaple, who are among the increasing numbers running successful day-care abortion centres. Costs, waiting time and workload could all be cut with expansion of this system, and the safety of early termination by the suction technique used for day-care is now proven and undisputed.

Professor Huntingford points out, 'At the moment it is costing the NHS about £5 million to perform just under half the abortions that are needed. If we put our minds to it we could provide all of them for not more than £3½ million.' With the cost of an out-patient abortion only £25 against £80, the current NHS estimate for a hospital abortion, he is obviously right.

Professor François Lafitte, chairman of BPAS, believes that the Health Service could cope with the whole annual demand for some 100 000 abortions (a figure likely to drop as contraceptive measures and sterilization provision improves) by setting up twelve or fifteen regional treatment centres, employing doctors part-time by the session, and offering day-care to up to half their patients. He adds, 'Had we a Minister bold enough to do that, BPAS would happily make him a free gift of our three treatment centres and our entire network of local counselling, pregnancy-testing and contraceptive advice centres.'

It is a good offer, but meanwhile it would be something if the DHSS backed Brook Clinics, BPAS and the other charities on abortion, as they already do on contraception and vasectomy with some financial support. Under the law all these services are supposed to be available and free. As yet they are not.

It might be well to add just a few comments from highly respected gynaecologists, made in 1977 when the Benyon Bill was threatening the present abortion law. It will happen again and their words should be remembered:

My experience has shown that the 1967 Abortion Act allows one to provide a humane and safe service for women.

RICHARD BEARD, *professor of obstetrics and gynaecology, St Mary's and Samaritan Hospital*

I feel particularly concerned for the reticent and inarticulate woman. It is the duty of the medical profession to provide help for those who most need it.

DR STUART CARNE, *treasurer, Royal College of General Practitioners, and senior lecturer, Postgraduate Medical School*

There is no doubt if the Benyon Bill were ever to become law it would seriously reduce the number of women who could obtain legal and safe abortions in this country.

DAVID PANTIN, *consultant obstetrician and gynaecologist, St Mary's Hospital, London*

The amending legislation White and Benyon have moved would result in later and more dangerous operations. Also, by separating nursing homes from referral agencies, it would eliminate the financial assistance which charities give women who cannot afford to pay.

DR MALCOLM POTTS, *consultant to International Planned Parenthood Association*

Malcolm Potts emphasized the most dangerous single aspect of the recent attempts to alter our abortion laws. It was proposed that a condition of licensing pregnancy advisory bureaux was that they should have no financial connection with abortion clinics. It sounds perhaps protective, but in effect would be destructive, as it would effectively prevent charities like BPAS from subsidizing abortions within their own clinics as they do now. This is often vital for women who cannot afford the fees nor get an NHS abortion, because they just happen to be in a restrictive area or under an anti-abortion doctor.

Future developments

All through this book I have tried not only to deal with currently
available treatments but to look ahead as well, and so this
chapter would not be complete without some mention of
prostaglandin suppositories.

For a long time this substance extracted from the prostate
gland, as the name implies, has been heralded as a possible
method of inducing termination in early pregnancy. In
December 1977 it was reported that Professor Bygdeman of
Stockholm had completed trials in which 200 women administered vaginal prostaglandin suppositories to themselves under
supervision of an outpatient clinic. All the women were in the
early part of pregnancy with only three weeks or less elapsed
since their last missed period. Complete and safe abortions
were produced in 97 per cent of the women and three-quarters
of the users of this trial method were confident enough to feel
they would be prepared to use it at home. Although Professor
Bygdeman still felt at the moment the method should only be
used with a degree of medical supervision he admitted that 'the
study opens the possibility that women could treat themselves,
which is something that may be developed in the future'.

Perhaps the real future lies, for the sake of conscience, convenience and comfort, in the regular use of a similar type of
preparation each month to bring on a period for all women
not wanting to conceive, so that they never even know if conception has occurred. Proved safe and effective after proper
trials had been carried out, such a method would inevitably
take a great deal of heat out of the whole abortion debate, a
great deal of anxiety out of women's lives, and could make
contraception as we know it now virtually obsolete.

8. Infertility

Ever since researching for this book, I have especially looked forward to writing this chapter. I have longed to report on what are perhaps the most exciting and successful advances in the whole medical field for women.

In recent years new medical and surgical techniques have pretty well doubled the chances of helping the infertile marriage. At present, the success rate is estimated at around 60 per cent, and there are even more hopeful developments just around the corner.

It has always been considered one of the basic human rights to have children, yet tragically there are over two million people in Britain alone, unsuccessfully striving to become parents. It's an irony that, while many find over-fertility a problem, others seem unable to achieve the longed-for family. About one couple in six have difficulty in conceiving and every week some 1600 people face up to the fact that they have a fertility problem.

More and more hospitals now are setting up special clinics for infertility, but the first step should be a talk with the family doctor. John Newton, the consultant gynaecologist who runs the famous Infertility Clinic at King's College Hospital, London, believes some couples rather jump the gun in self-diagnosing the problem too soon.

These days there is a tendency to expect everything to be instant and planned. Couples expect planned contraception followed by planned fertility just when they want it. It doesn't always work like that. No couple should consider consulting their doctor until they have been trying to conceive for at least six to nine months without result. After a preliminary talk with their GP, probably a further three to six months should be allowed before the decision to consult a gynaecologist.

Once this decision is made, the most thorough investigations are undertaken to determine the cause, and it is very important to have the cooperation of the husband in this. Although infertility has traditionally been blamed on the woman, modern medical knowledge has proved that female disorders actually account for only about one third of conception problems. Another third involve purely male factors and the remainder can be a joint problem.

It is understandable that in the past some men were sometimes reluctant to come forward for the necessary check-up, simply because of the age-old confusion between virility and infertility. Anything which might be a reflection on their 'machismo' was unacceptable, and this is still the attitude among some West Indian men. Roman Catholic men are also often unwilling, though for the very different reason that they believe supplying sperm for investigation must involve masturbation, considered a sin by their church.

The male investigation

A specimen of semen freshly donated by masturbation is preferred as the most accurate method of checking what is called the sperm count, and also for determining if sufficient sperm are healthy and active. Special tactful arrangements for complete privacy are made for men willing and able to do this while at the clinic.

But for the man who really cannot cope with this method either at the clinic or at home, another way is to withdraw at the vital moment during normal intercourse and ejaculate into a dry, wide-mouthed jar kept ready beside the bed. However it is obtained, the semen must be received at the laboratory and examined within two hours for accurate results.

Yet a third alternative method is called the post-coital test. This is carried out on the wife but must be done within six hours of having intercourse. The doctor takes a specimen from the cervix which still contains semen, assuming coitus has been correctly undertaken. So in a sense this way is also a check on that aspect, but it is rather more difficult to accurately assess the quality of the sperm.

That, of course, is the whole point of these tests, because if the problem lies there it is useless to subject the woman to the far more difficult and complex tests needed to check on female infertility.

Gynaecologists, and for that matter family doctors consulted in the early stages, really like to see a couple together. Often quite simple things can lie at the root of the trouble and I was amazed to be told by John Newton, a recognized expert in this field, that often just the current fashion for tight underpants and tight jeans can encourage male infertility by raising the temperature of the testicles. So those tight sexy male outfits are paradoxically anti-fertility symbols, at least at the strictly medical level.

The doctor will, of course, also want to ask about general health and about specific illness which may affect fertility, such as mumps which can damage the testicles or gonorrhoea which may damage the vas deferens, the tube down which the sperm pass. He may also ask about smoking or drinking, as an excess of either can reduce sperm production as well as frequency of intercourse.

A fertile man should have around 200 million sperm in each ejaculation and dealing in that sort of number obviously no one is going to count them one by one. What happens when a sperm count is taken is that a drop of semen is placed under a high-powered microscope. The number of sperm seen is then related to the known volume of semen under view and this enables an accurate count to be worked out. It may prove to be just a little below normal or it may be very low indeed. Sometimes, though very rarely, there are no sperm present at all and in such cases sadly nothing can be done to help the man directly, unless the ejaculate is being diverted into the bladder, which sometimes occurs after prostate operations.

The sperm are also checked under the microscope to see that sufficient of them are normal and active. Figures of 75 per cent normal and 70 per cent active are the kind often quoted as being acceptable. But with all these factors it is important to remember the effect on fertility is only going to be relative. A lower sperm count only means a lower chance of conception; it does not mean total infertility. The same applies to lower numbers of active and normal sperm. Obviously the larger the numbers of strong and active sperm, the better the chance each time of one of them not only making that long swim to meet the egg, but having the strength to penetrate on contact.

In this respect there can be one other important factor. Sometimes the woman's vaginal mucus can be hostile to the sperm, often in the sense that it is thicker than normal and so presents a more difficult barrier to penetrate. To check on this, the post-coital test would need to be carried out between six and twenty hours after intercourse.

All these things must be checked before the appropriate treatment can be determined, and the investigation for the woman is even more extensive.

The female investigation

Mr Joe Jordan, consultant gynaecologist at Birmingham Woman's Hospital and at Birmingham Maternity Hospital, described to me how he likes to proceed with his infertility patients.

I prefer to see the couple together and of course carry out the tests to exclude any male infertility as you've described. If the man won't cooperate in the early stages, then I must press ahead and get all the information I can from the wife. In any case I like to have a good talk with her and get a full history. It is the whole woman we are investigating, and so I want to know about general health and again about any diseases which in her case may cause tubal blockage, such as pelvic inflammation, gonorrhoea or a previous ectopic pregnancy, that is where a fertilized egg has implanted in the tube not the womb.

I also need to know about regularity of intercourse and of menstruation, and whether there is mid-cycle pain or dysmenorrhoea [painful periods], both of which can suggest ovulation. I go on to do a full physical check-up, of course, with pelvic examination, breasts and also X-ray of chest and skull.

Mr Jordan emphasized that perhaps the most vital tests were blood tests to establish hormone levels, including that of the thyroid where imbalance either way, too much or too little, can sometimes affect fertility.

Obviously the levels of both female sex hormones are highly relevant, and so it is helpful if the visit to the gynaecologist can be arranged in the second half of the cycle, as the important pregnancy hormone, progesterone, only comes into the picture then.

'If hormone problems can be excluded,' Mr Jordan went on, 'the next job is to make sure the tubes down which the egg must pass are clear. This used to involve blowing carbon dioxide through or using a dye in conjunction with X-rays and both these methods are still used. But more often we use a laparoscope which usually enables us to see all we want.'

Treatment and male infertility

The sort of treatment given is obviously going to depend on the cause or causes for infertility which investigations may reveal. Even if the problem proves to involve the man, very often the gynaecologist will undertake the treatment required, or sometimes refer instead to a urologist (a doctor specializing in the urinary tract) or to one of the new infertility clinics for men. Ten years ago these simply did not exist, but now many hospitals run them, often in conjunction with their main infertility clinic.

Treatment for the man may vary from a simple change in smoking or drinking habits or wearing looser clothing, to minor surgery to cure varicose veins, which can occur round the vas deferens and sometimes interfere with fertility. But more often it will be a matter of trying to improve the number or quality of the sperm.

This can often be achieved with drugs and many doctors have reported clomiphene, one of the mild fertility drugs used to treat female infertility, as also effective in improving sperm count in men. This acts on the pituitary gland to increase hormone production.

The most commonly used drug in this country, and one with a good success record in treating sub-fertility, is a natural male hormone, commercially known as Pro-viron. This only came on the scene in 1971, and it has the great advantage of not depressing the man's own natural hormone production, as other hormone products tend to do, so cancelling out any gain. Trials with Pro-viron at Chelsea Hospital for Women found that one in five women whose husbands were treated with this drug because of low sperm count became pregnant.[23]

Where the sperm count does not respond to drug treatment, doctors have yet another trick up their sleeves these days. It has proved possible and very often successful to pool 'split ejaculates'. That inelegant but graphic phrase means exactly what it says. It means putting together from several separate ejaculations the first part, known to contain the most sperm. Providing the semen is frozen quickly it can be kept until enough has been obtained. In this concentrated form a good sperm count can be built up. Then at mid-cycle when ovulation takes place, the husband's sperm is introduced around the cervix by simply injecting it well up into the vagina. This is known as AIH, or artificial insemination by husband. AID, artificial insemination by donor, uses sperm from an anonymous source and this is discussed later. It would obviously only be used in the event of no success being achieved with the husband's own sperm and where both husband and wife agree.

Treatment of female infertility

Where this is found to be due to infrequent ovulation or complete lack of ovulation, a great deal can now be done to help in the great majority of cases.

The big break through came back in 1961 with successful use of what have come to be called 'the infertility drugs'. Carl Gemzell and his team of Swedish doctors at Upsala were first in the field, but almost simultaneously the same hormones were isolated and put into successful use here in Britain at Birmingham Women's Hospital.[24]

It had been known for some time that what are called gonadotrophins, taken from animals, could sometimes prod sluggish human ovaries into action. Gonadotrophic hormones are the ones we have already met – FHS or follicle stimulating hormone and LH or luteinizing hormone. In Chapter 2 we saw how these hormones secreted by the pituitary gland cause the dormant egg cells in the ovaries to ripen and finally the follicle to burst each month releasing an egg.

Hormones obtained from animals can sometimes work extremely well. Insulin, used to treat diabetes, was originally obtained from the pancreas of pigs, and Premarin, one of the oestrogens most widely used to treat the menopause is extracted from the urine of pregnant mares, both utilized with few problems. But with the animal gonadotrophins there proved to be unacceptable risks, involving responses from the human rejection mechanism with antibodies being formed, which could sometimes result in severe shock and even death.

So the hunt was on, throughout the world, to find a way of extracting human gonadotrophins and making them do the same job but safely. At Birmingham Women's Hospital, Dr Carl Crook, an endocrinologist (a specialist in hormones) together with Professor Wilfred Butt, a biochemist, and Mr Logan-Edwards, a gynaecologist, working as a team achieved the first successful births in this country with the aid of human gonadotrophins.

It was an exciting achievement with none of the problems that had been associated with the animal extracts. But in the early days before the crucial nature of the dosage of FSH and LH to be used was properly understood and controlled, the ovaries sometimes got prodded a bit too fiercely, producing not just one egg or even two but sometimes a whole lot at once, which led to the much publicized multiple births. Now, however, treatment is carefully tailored to each individual woman and the rise in oestrogen which the drugs produce is carefully monitored. In this way multiple births are almost entirely avoided except for a higher than normal ratio of twins.

At King's College clinic they actually aim at twins, believing that the dosage likely to ripen two eggs at a time gives a better chance of pregnancy. Some women who have waited perhaps many years for a baby are only too happy for the chance to achieve a family in one go. Of the 1000 new patients seen there every year with fertility problems, a quarter will have failure of ovulation and some will need gonadotrophins. John Newton, in charge of their clinic, explained to me how their close monitoring system works with this treatment.

If the rate at which the oestrogen rises is excessively steep, then we know the patient is at risk of too many eggs being released and perhaps fertilized. So every day a blood sample is analysed and, if necessary, we stop treatment and tell the patient not to have intercourse until everything has settled down again. In two or three weeks we can start again with an adjusted dosage.

As will be obvious by now, the use of the human gonado-trophins still requires very careful supervision and control, and they are also rather expensive. In many women failure to ovulate can be overcome by another less complicated and less expensive substance called clomiphene, and tests can be done to indicate if response is likely to this simpler treatment.

The man who played a major part in the development of clomiphene is Robert Greenblatt, one of the world's leading endocrinologists and a very good friend and adviser to me. The preparation is not in itself a hormone but what is termed an anti-oestrogen. It works by suppressing oestrogen, which causes the pituitary to step up production of FSH and LH to try and prod the ovaries into producing more oestrogen. This happens naturally as women approach the menopause, and these days high levels of FSH are accepted as an indicator of the onset of the change of life.

When oestrogen is artificially suppressed by clomiphene, the same mechanism goes into action with increased production of FSH and LH, and in the younger woman this may revive ovulation. Because it works further back in the chain of events and results in production of her own gonadotrophins, there is very little problem of over-stimulation and multiple births.

Yet another drug is being increasingly used to treat infer-tility in cases where tests reveal high levels of another hormone called prolactin. This is the hormone which stimulates breast milk and at the same time interrupts ovulation, which is why women who are breast-feeding are usually safe from pregnancy. Unfortunately in just a few women prolactin seems to be kept at a high level and works to suppress ovulation all the time. Bromocriptine tablets replace a missing brain chemical which normally controls prolactin production, and so checks un-wanted milk production and restarts ovulation.

At St Mary's Hospital in London, where considerable success is being achieved with this new and powerful drug, endocrino-logist Howard Jacobs emphasized that, because bromocriptine acts on the brain, each patient must first be carefully screened and X-rays done to preclude a tumour, which can occasionally underlie raised prolactin. Dr Jacobs is optimistic about the treatment.

I believe bromocriptine may eventually replace gonadotrophin treatment in many cases, as it has the great advantage of merely removing a common cause of failure to ovulate and allowing the patient's own natural hormone levels to operate and her own natural ovulation cycle to take over. If we can prove it is safe, some 40 000 infertile women might benefit.

Bromocriptine also works for another group of women whose prolactin levels are not high, yet they still fail to get pregnant. Their problems seem to be related to low levels of progesterone in the second half of the cycle, when normally higher levels of this hormone should be at work. In a way not fully understood, bromocriptine appears able to correct this.

Ian Cooke, professor of gynaecology and obstetrics at Sheffield University who runs an infertility unit at the Jessop Hospital there, told me:

In the first instance in women who are not ovulating and where prolactin levels appear normal, we would use clomiphene. If that fails we go on to the gonadotrophins in those cases, but where pro-lactin is high we certainly use bromocriptine. It also seems to work for others who appear to ovulate but can't get pregnant, and it does it in some way through raising progesterone just after ovulation. We are getting a third of all our infertility cases, where we can find no obvious cause for the problem, conceiving on bromocriptine.

So in suitable cases the present range of infertility treatments offers real hope, but even that is not the end of the story. From Mr Ted Logan-Edwards, who was in at what might appro-priately be termed the birth of the first generation of fertility drugs, I learned of future developments.

The next generation of fertility drugs are likely to be even better. We have already gone further back in the chain of events by using drugs which stimulate the hypothalamus and pituitary to actually produce the gonadotrophins in such a way that the balance and amount natural for each individual woman is achieved. Now we are going back even one step further still, with the use of what is called Releasing Hormone, which releases the hormone which stimulates the pituitary into producing the gonadotrophins which prod the ovary to secrete the oestrogen.

Although it all sounds a bit like that old nursery rhyme, 'The House that Jack Built', the logic is clear. 'The further back we are able to influence events in the chain,' Mr Logan-Edwards pointed out, 'the more natural is the later sequence of events leading to the vital ovulation.

'The problem with Releasing Hormone is that pure RH, as it is called, has been difficult to extract,' he warned, 'and this has made it expensive to use. Now, however, RH has been synthesized in the laboratory and there is more hope for wider usage with time.'

The other cause for infertility already mentioned, where the woman's cervical mucus is hostile to the sperm, often because it is too thick, can usually be successfully treated with oestrogen, which seems to thin it down. Sometimes artificial insemination with the husband's sperm has to be resorted to, if oestrogen alone does not overcome the problem.

The other main cause of infertility in women is nothing to do with hormone levels and is a mechanical problem. Some 20 per cent of infertile women prove to have blocked or partially blocked fallopian tubes, preventing free passage of the egg and any meeting with the sperm to have even a chance of fertilization.

As Mr Jordan mentioned, a test still often used to check on this consists of blowing carbon dioxide gas through the tubes. Called tubal insufflation, it is normally done under a general anaesthetic and the doctor can see on a graph attached to the apparatus whether one or both tubes are blocked, or he may listen with a stethoscope. Some doctors believe this method may even help to clear the tubes.

A test more often used today in conjunction with a laparoscope, and/or X-rays, involves injection of a dye, which should travel the length of the tube if it is not blocked.

If both tubes are found to be blocked tubal surgery may be recommended. The surgeon removes the blocked portion and rejoins the tube. It is not such a difficult procedure but the success rate is not as high as might be expected, largely because scar tissue often forms to reblock the tube yet again. At one time the chances of successful surgery was only between 10 and 20 per cent, but development of delicate micro-surgical techniques has considerably improved on that.

Also at Hammersmith Hospital in London, Robert Winston has successfully carried out complete fallopian transplants. So far this has only been done with animals, but if and when it can be applied to human patients, it will offer hope to women where normal tubal surgery has failed.

But another exciting method is also being pioneered which by-passes the whole fallopian system. This work has brought what the popular press calls the 'test-tube baby' very close indeed.

Oldham gynaecologist P. C. Steptoe, the man who first pioneered laparoscope techniques, has also pioneered much of this work in conjunction with Dr Robert Edwards, a physiologist at Cambridge.

If you saw the excellent BBC 'Horizon' programme on infertility called 'A Child of Your Own', written and produced by Christopher Riley, you may have seen this amazing process known as *in vitro* fertilization. *In vitro* simply means 'in glass' and the egg is fertilized outside the body literally in a glass dish, which is where the concept of a test-tube baby comes in.

But first gonadotrophins are administered to the mother so that what is called super-ovulation is achieved with several eggs ripening at once. Then using a laparoscope the surgeon sucks out from the ovaries the biggest and most hopeful-looking follicles.

If they are found to contain the hoped-for eggs these are placed one to a glass dish, each of which already contains pools of active male sperm donated by the husband. Within a few hours, in 70 per cent of cases, one of the milling sperm manages to penetrate an egg and cell division begins.

There is a danger with this sort of brief description (as with the condensation of the process necessary for the 'Horizon' film version) that it could all be made to appear too easy. In fact, it is work that can only be attempted by highly specialized teams and it is by no means widely available yet. To begin with, the surgeons are dealing with the recovery and attempted fertilization of human eggs too small to be seen by the naked eye. Fine micro-surgery has to be used but equally delicate and crucial, if there is to be any chance of success, is the timing factor at each stage.

First the egg sac and content must have reached just the right critical stage in the monthly ripening process; the sperm must also be mature and what is termed 'capacitated' so that it has the power to penetrate the egg. Most important of all, however, is the final stage of implanting the fertilized egg back into the woman, the development of the egg must be absolutely synchronized with the development of the uterine lining which will also have been going ahead.

This is complicated by the fact that the initial surgery to extract the egg from the ovary (even the minor laparoscope technique) can be enough, in conjunction with use of anaesthetic, to upset the mother's normal hormonal pattern and progression. A further complicating factor is that the normal development rate of the tiny embryo, which inside the mother's body would keep pace with development of the uterine lining, tends to be slowed down *in vitro*. Both these influences contribute to the problem of keeping egg and uterine lining 'in sync', and almost certainly explains why up until now successful implantation in humans eluded the highly skilled teams at work to solve infertility by methods already used successfully in animals. For there lies the irony. In the animal breeding world, fertilization *in vitro* and re-implantation is being successfully and increasingly widely used now to achieve super stock without endangering the female. Top Charolais cows, for instance, are treated with a fertility drug to induce 'super-ovulation'. With animals surgery is not even required to recover the ripening eggs: they are simply flushed out and fertilized *in vitro* with sperm from a super bull. But they are not implanted back in the Charolais female. Instead they are injected around the cervix of *ordinary* cows, whose cycle has been synchronized exactly with that of the female Charolais by giving both animals injections of prostaglandin. These pre-natal 'adoptive mothers' accept the eggs, gestate them, and finally give birth, not to ordinary calves but to super-calves, the true offspring of the super-Charolais and the super-bull who contributed the genetic packages, the donor egg and donor sperm.

This is breeding for success with a vengeance and, if it were not for the objections of the Jockey Club who would lose enormous stud fees, the same system could equally be applied to horses. There is every possibility that by using the same technique and introducing the egg from one woman, fertilizing *in vitro*, and implanting it in the body of another, with both cycles carefully synchronized, the present problems of implantation could be overcome or at least reduced. But what is ethical and acceptable with animals becomes a different matter with humans and human feelings to be considered.

Doctors working in this area of research accept that using pre-natal foster mothers, who would not have suffered the trauma of previous surgery to recover the eggs, would greatly increase chances of successful implantation, but they also feel the ethical and legal problems involved are too great to justify such a step.

Using donor eggs given by a willing volunteer to help an infertile woman who can give birth normally but cannot ovulate, offers a slightly less traumatic alternative and again would have a very good chance of working. Many doctors feel there is really little difference between using donor eggs and donor sperm. There is a difference, however, in the way in which they have to be obtained, and a woman donating eggs would have to face the minor discomfort and minor risk of laparoscope surgery just to help another woman.

The pioneer of *in vitro* fertilization and implantation, Mr P. C. Steptoe, can conceive of just one set of circumstances in which he might undertake such an operation.

It could just be ethically and emotionally acceptable within the confines of a close, loving and well-adjusted family. There's not really much difference logically between accepting a donor egg and accepting donor sperm. One can imagine perhaps a fertile sister prepared for the right reasons to donate an egg, or even bear a child, to overcome insuperable infertility problems in a less fortunate sister.

In fact, as so often, the technical problems are likely to be easier to solve than the ethical ones. Successful implantation will soon cease to be a hit-or-miss affair and become routine. Even since I started researching the subject a few months ago things have moved fast. Success in freezing donor eggs now offers the opportunity of storing them and attempting implantation in successive cycles. This not only offers *more* chances but *better* chances during later cycles after the mother's hormone patterns, disturbed by the initial surgery, have had a chance to settle down.

The team working at St Thomas's Hospital under gynaecologist Ian Ferguson have also been on the trail of a special protein which may be involved in successful implantation. But Ian Ferguson told me very recently:

We now also pin even more hope on direct implantation into the fallopian tubes. This involves needle puncture and micro-tubal surgery, but it's possible the tubal environment itself may well have some influence on successful implantation. It is obviously only possible where some remnant of tube remains and it does have the advantage of temporarily opening that up. In at least one case, although the *in vitro* fertilized egg did not implant, a subsequent normally fertilized egg succeeded in getting through the newly opened bit of tube and a pregnancy resulted.

Where no vestige of tube remains available for this method the St Thomas's team are now using direct implantation into the uterus itself; Ian Ferguson explained, 'This at least avoids the risk of ectopic pregnancy involved when introducing the egg through the cervix or into tubal remnant.'

In fact, up until the present day, the only absolutely documented success with implantation was sadly an ectopic pregnancy, reported in the medical literature by gynaecologist Patrick Steptoe. It came as no surprise to many when Mr Steptoe finally achieved his goal, with the triumphant birth of a baby daughter to Lesley and John Brown on 25 July 1978. It is vital that, in time, the exposure they and their baby received in the press will not prove harmful, and that they will have the opportunity of leading a normal life. Otherwise, there is a real fear that the medical ranks will be promptly closed. In any event, one hopes that this historic birth will become a symbol to thousands of infertile women of what the future can hold for them.

If I seem to have given a lot of space to these science-fiction developments which are so rapidly becoming science-fact, it is because all of us have to start thinking, while there is still time, just how far and how fast we want them to go.

There is another even more seemingly way-out method of reproduction which just in the last two years has begun to emerge as a practical possibility. It is not likely to be offered to any woman as a means of solving infertility in the near future, or even applied to the human race within the next decade or so, but it has been shown to be possible with other warm-blooded mammals, and that means it could eventually be done with man.

Cloning

This is a method of duplicating life, of producing identical carbon copies of living creatures, without any mating process, any mix of genetic material or, indeed, any 'parents' at all.

Cloning comes from the Greek word for 'cuttings' and it is a vegetative process now to be applied to animals. The chapter on conception explained that, while normal body cells contain a full set of chromosomes, the egg cell of the female and the sperm of the male each contain only a half-set, so that when they fuse the full complement is achieved. Once this happens the egg cell recognizes the presence of all the genetic information it needs to produce a new life and starts to divide.

With cloning, the ordinary nucleus of the female egg with its half-set of chromosomes is destroyed by irradiation. Using delicate micro-surgery, into the now empty egg cell is placed the nucleus of an adult cell of the same species, male or female but containing a full set of chromosomes like all body cells.

The female egg cell senses the presence of the full set of chromosomes and, fooled into thinking it has been fertilized, it starts to divide and grow. But the new life that has been so ingeniously and deviously triggered, owes nothing to the female egg except for protection and nourishment. The actual genetic material comes *only* from the nucleus of the body cell inserted into it, and so the growing embryo is simply a carbon copy, identical in every detail to the animal from which the body cell was taken.

Until 1975 it had only proved possible to do this with the large eggs of cold-blooded frogs. But in that year, Dr Derek Bromhall, a British scientist working on a Nuffield grant at Oxford, showed the technique could be adapted to rabbits, warm-blooded animals whose eggs – only the size of a speck of dust – are no bigger than those of humans.[25] So carbon-copy people became technically possible.

Dr Bromhall himself is emphatic that he wants no part in any extension of his work toward cloning people. 'No one in their right mind would clone humans,' he insists.

While cloning could be used to reproduce rare human genius and compassion, to benefit the world by ensuring more future Einsteins, Mozarts or Madame Curies, it could equally and rather more likely be abused to duplicate monsters, tyrants and warlords.

It may sound like futuristic nonsense but it is taken very seriously by many scientists including Gordon Rattray Taylor, himself a trained biologist. In his best-seller, *The Biological Time Bomb*, he speculated that cloning could be used not only to produce vast carbon-copy armies of specially aggressive individuals, but also and horrifically to clone submissive or even subnormal people to become a slave race.

On the other hand, as even Dr Bromhall admits, there are wonderful possibilities in cloning if it is confined to agriculture. 'It could cut out all random chance associated with normal breeding techniques,' he explained. 'With cloning you could take a top cow and produce exact replicas to propagate any desirable characteristic you wanted, such as exceptional milk yield.'

He is even more enthusiastic about possible spin-off from his work which could give real insight into how cancer cells differ from normal cells. 'My work with cloning involved transferring the nucleus of cells,' he pointed out, 'and from this we might be able to find out if the carcinogenic factor in cancer cells is contained in the nucleus or in the other part of the cell.'

In developing and above all controlling the exciting new technology, nothing is going to be simple, and medicine and science which can alter the shape of our lives and our world is perhaps too important to be left just to doctors or to scientists. Society, and that means *us*, must share in the difficult ethical decisions that are going to have to be made – about donor eggs, pre-natal fostering, cloning and also about genetic engineering, which before the end of this century may offer the chance of replacing faulty genes, creating new forms of life and could lead to Superman or super disaster.

Well, after that irresistible diversion into such fascinating and controversial future developments, there are still legal and ethical problems to be considered with currently used techniques.

Artificial insemination by husband (AIH)

This has already been mentioned earlier in this chapter and providing both partners agree there are few ethical problems. Under existing law any child conceived in this way is presumed to be legitimate, unless the husband can prove he is not the father. AIH is available under the NHS.

Artificial insemination by donor (AID)

So too is AID, though there can be long waiting lists. At King's College Hospital Infertility Clinic the waiting list for this particular service is twelve months at the moment. The donor, of course, is anonymous but guaranteed healthy. From details on the records he is matched as closely as possible to the husband both physically and intellectually. This is very important to help the child to be fully accepted, and it is even more important in these cases that the husband should himself be convinced that he *wants* a child to be born to his wife by this means – he must not be over-persuaded, emotionally black-mailed or bludgeoned into agreement because of any sense of guilt about his own sperm being unsuitable. Indeed the reason may lie in the joint problem of the cervical mucus of his wife being hostile to his particular sperm.

One rather subtle way some doctors use is to mix husband's sperm and donor sperm together, which leaves at least a slight chance, in theory if not in practice, that the one sperm to penetrate could after all have come from the husband.

In law, the situation is not yet very satisfactory, and a child born by AID sometimes may not be considered legitimate until the parents legally adopt it. A panel of doctors has recommended legitimacy laws should be extended to cover the AID child, but nothing has yet been done.

For the woman, of course, providing the marital relationship is basically strong, AID offers a good solution, giving her the experience of carrying and bearing a child which at least inherits her own half of the genetic package.

The accident of genes, chromosomes and genetic mix, are far less important in forging a relationship between parents and a child than are the long hours of care, tenderness and love built up over the years. So there is every chance that the bond between an AID baby and its father can be just as good (or just as bad) as between any other child and its *natural* father. One can imagine the temptation, however, if things at any point go badly with an AID child, to brood or bicker about where undesirable traits have come from. In even the best of marriages it's not unknown for a father to complain bitterly to the mother about '*your* child', but to boast complacently about '*our* child' when all is going well. The mother can often employ the same tactics in reverse, but with an AID baby it could be a touchy area, which is precisely why it is not something to be undertaken within a fragile marriage or offered to an unstable or immature couple.

Having said this, it is perhaps only fair to add that *Doctor* magazine in March 1978 reported happy and satisfied AID parents returning to ask for a second or third child, so that obviously for the right people it works well.

Dr Louis Hughes, who works from London's Royal Free Hospital and was the first man in Britain to set up a sperm bank was quoted as saying 'It is proving a very happy procedure with very gratifying results.' His donors are medical students at the Royal Free, and there is no problem in finding donors and matching physical characteristics to the husbands, including body build, height, hair colour and eye colour. If the wife is rhesus negative, a rhesus negative donor is used to avoid complications. If the husband has obvious Jewish looks, Dr Hughes will find a Jewish donor, but otherwise not. 'By and large, genes don't carry religion,' was Dr Hughes's comment.

The greatest problem is apparently with Asian couples, where having a child can be of great importance, and yet Asian donors are rare. All donors, of course, as at Kings College and other centres, are screened for medical and family history. 'I would not use anyone with diabetes or Huntingdon's chorea', Dr Hughes added and he pointed out that using medical students also had the advantage of their understanding the importance of *not* being a donor if they were suffering from a genital discharge and could pass on VD.

But medical problems are easier to overcome than legal ones or ethical ones. Doctors could act as their own donors and would then know where their genetic offspring were. Then there is the question of AID being provided to lesbian couples. Society has to do a great deal of thinking on all these matters, ancient laws have to be updated, and once again doctors must not be left to bear all the responsibility and make all the decisions.

Donor eggs

As discussed, this development is already a practical possibility, and once the implantation problems are fully solved many infertile women could be helped by receiving donor eggs. With the husband's sperm used, it is the woman who would have to come to terms with the fact that the female half of the genetic package had been supplied by some other woman. Again, despite Mr Steptoe's feeling that it would be more ethical within a close-knit family, there could actually be good argument for anonymity, as with male donor sperm, providing similar careful matching techniques were employed.

The reverse process, strictly equivalent to the pre-natal foster-mother cow bringing the Charolais calf to term, is not likely ever to be acceptable in human terms. One can imagine few women prepared to go through the nine months and face the pain and trauma of childbirth, only then to hand over the baby to the donor mother, who was able to supply the egg fertilized by her own husband, but for some reason could not gestate or give birth. Certainly no responsible doctors or medical teams would be likely to undertake supervision of such a scheme but it's not impossible to conceive of pirate baby hatcheries. Of course some young women might be prepared to act as pre-natal foster mothers if the money was good enough, and there are always unfortunately unscrupulous operators ready to make fortunes out of the greed of some and the despair of others. It could foreshadow an Aldous Huxley 'Brave New World' concept, against which future generations may need to be on guard.

Artificial wombs

The test-tube baby or the cloned embryo will really come into its own if the work being done round the world to produce artificial wombs or artificial placenta ever succeeds. So far, despite vast sums being spent particularly in America and Russia, no one has managed to overcome the problem of keeping the blood supply to the foetus clear of waste products. Lamb foetuses have been kept alive for a day or two, but that is as far as it has gone, and perhaps we should be relieved.

Although the work is strictly directed toward means of keeping very premature embryos alive, it could like so many scientific techniques be abused. While the *New Scientist* magazine stated firmly that 'the development of the perfect artificial placenta can only be a matter of time', one of our own leading experts is not optimistic. Geoffrey Chamberlain, consultant gynaecologist at Queen Charlotte's and Chelsea Women's Hospitals in London, told me: 'A matter of time in my view still means a long time. It needs such vast resources to crack this one that, for the moment, we have given up work in this country.'

So the real test-tube baby, never knowing the security of a mother's womb, is still a long way off and thank goodness. But the embryo fertilized outside the body and re-implanted is already a reality at the time this book goes to press.

Coming to terms with infertility

With so many new techniques, it is in some ways even harder for the woman desperately wanting a child to have to come to terms with the fact that none of the methods will work for her.

But that can still be the situation for quite a few couples. There is an estimated 40 per cent where no medical reason can be discovered.

There is absolutely no evidence that couples unable to have children have any more psycho-sexual problems than others, but because of their frustrated wish to have children they obviously question this area of their lives more closely and worry about it more.

It may well be worth seeking advice if there is any possibility that the trouble could lie with infrequent intercourse, which obviously reduces the chances of conception, or with premature ejaculation or insufficient penetration. Fear of pain on the woman's part, or lack of preliminary love play leading to frigidity can also play a part. A retroverted or tipped uterus can make conception more difficult, but this is usually over-come by the woman lying on her abdomen with hips supported by a pillow for half an hour after intercourse in order to place the cervical opening in contact with the gathering sperm. A rear entry position for coitus can also help. A tipped uterus would, of course be normally discovered on the first consultation with a gynaecologist, assuming the couple had already tackled medical aspects of infertility.

It is often less easy for a man than for a woman to discuss possible sexual factors, because of the wretched lingering and totally wrong association between infertility and implied lack of virility.

But for both a man and a woman the growing realization that they will probably never have children can be bitter particu-larly after all checks and treatments have been tried. The great thing that has to be fought is any feeling of inadequacy, loss of value or being 'different' and cut off from the great fulfilled majority. Gaps can open up between the childless couple and their friends with growing families as interests diverge, and the position is never made easier by the tactless unthinking ques-tion, 'Have you any children?' which is so often an innocent conversational gambit with strangers. Then there can be recriminations at home with mothers and mothers-in-law waiting for and wanting grandchildren.

Anger against oneself or one's partner, depression and over-sensitivity are all common reactions to infertility, building to a climax in the thirties age-group when hope really begins to fade after years of going the rounds and finding no answer.

These days there is no easy solution in adoption as there once was for many couples. Free contraceptive services, their avail-ability to the unmarried and hopefully a greater sense of responsibility in sexual relationships are combining not only to reduce the number of illegitimate births, abortions and con-ceptions before marriage, but all these things taken together are drastically reducing the number of babies available for adoption. There has been a fall of nearly a quarter in extra-marital conceptions for example among women aged sixteen to nineteen between the years 1972 and 1976, with a corresponding decline in the twenty to twenty-four age group.

Of course there will always be coloured children, disabled children and a proportion of older children needing adoption for those able to accept the challenge this can represent. Short term fostering can be a way of channelling parental instinct for just a few people but it requires a special kind of loving, able to let go, and able to face the insecurity of never knowing when the moment will come for the child to be returned to its own home.

In 1977 a superb, practical booklet was written on this whole subject by Peter and Diane Houghton, who have been through it all and are able to give unsentimental constructive help. It is called *Unfocused Grief* and details are given in the recommended reading at the back. They wrote the booklet following a big meeting of childless couples held in Birmingham, which led to the formation of the National Association of the Childless. The aim of the association is not only to try and improve provision of treatment for infertility, but also to improve adoption and fostering services, and to gain acceptance of the childless (not least by themselves) as valuable members of society with special contributions to make.

There is no single solution but there is a way forward, and this booklet can certainly help it to be found more quickly and, perhaps, with less pain. There are compensations in the freedom, in the opportunity to develop your own personality and talents, to travel, even to develop substitute parental roles – but the approach must be positive and the discovery gradual. In the end everyone must find their own solution and the confidence to see that their lives are of value to themselves and to others.

9. Pregnancy and labour

Any woman pregnant for the first time, or even hoping to become pregnant for the first time, will have such a vital and personal interest in these fascinating subjects that she may well want really detailed information. Excellent books are available giving a detailed account of each phase of pregnancy and labour, and I have listed some at the back.

In this chapter I am going to deal briefly with the overall facts, but also put the emphasis on the new techniques and medical advances which are helping to make pregnancy and labour easier and safer and the babies produced healthier.

The early chemical pregnancy test based on detecting the rise in the hormone HCG (human chorionic gonadotrophin), which follows immediately on pregnancy has already been mentioned. Of course, for the woman who really wants a baby, there is no great urgency and the old-fashioned visit to her own doctor following a missed period may well suffice.

Your doctor will be happy to carry out the first examination quite early on within a few weeks of the first missed period. It enables him then to check the uterus before it becomes palpably enlarged and also to ensure not only that pregnancy has occurred but that the fertilized egg has implanted in the right place – actually in the uterus.

Ectopic pregnancy

Ectopic means literally 'in the wrong place', and is the medical term applied to a pregnancy outside the womb, usually within the fallopian tubes.

Normally the egg is fertilized within the tube, but wafted down to implant safely and securely in the uterus. Just very occasionally the fertilized egg may get caught up in a small pocket or have its passage slowed down because the tube is narrow or partially blocked. When this happens it may implant in the wall of the tube, which of course cannot expand sufficiently as the egg grows. This still usually leads to a missed period (or sometimes an abnormal one) and there may be some pain in the lower abdomen or vaginal bleeding. If an ectopic pregnancy is allowed to proceed it may end in the tube rupturing and so it is always very important to have this first check-up to ensure all is well.

The check-up, by your doctor is quite painless and involves a brief internal examination and gentle pressure on the abdomen at the same time, so that the shape of the uterus can be felt. Usually a smear test is also taken to ensure the vagina and cervix are healthy.

False or phantom pregnancy

In just a very few mysterious cases an imaginary or pseudo-pregnancy occurs. Nearly always the woman has desperately wanted a child for years, but the amazing thing is that the real physical signs of pregnancy may be convincingly reproduced. She may cease to menstruate, develop early morning nausea and even vomiting, while breasts become tender and enlarged with some pigmentation round the nipples. All these are signs and symptoms of real pregnancy, and it's a fascinating illustration of how closely mind and body are connected that all these physical changes can stem from a mental delusion.

In the past, before modern diagnostic methods, some women fooled themselves (and their doctors) right to the point of phantom labour too, which of course had no end product. It was all pretty sad and today the chemical pregnancy test, and another marvellous device called ultra sound can both be used to help convince the patient of the truth – that it was just in the mind.

Ultrasound

Most big hospitals now are equipped with special ultrasound machines which can detect both a healthy pregnancy or an ectopic pregnancy very early on. They work by a sort of radar system which uses ultrasonic echo-sounding waves of very high frequency which are beamed into the womb. They then form a picture shown on a fluorescent screen rather like TV. Ultrasound is not only extremely useful in the early stages if there is any possibility of an ectopic pregnancy (which always requires immediate surgery) but it also enables monitoring for growth rate and position of the foetus throughout pregnancy. Use of special ultrasound effects can also record pulsation and heart action actually within the living foetus, from about the thirteenth week of pregnancy onwards, which is much earlier than ordinary methods allow.

It is also extremely useful in later pregnancy, where there may be special reason for considering induction, and it has become a valuable way of checking that the baby is mature enough to be born safely. In the past sometimes calculations based on the last period could be wrong, and babies were induced who were too premature. Ultrasound is far more precise – health and maturity of the foetus can actually be *seen*, and it avoids the use of X-rays, which can be harmful if employed too often. The use of ultrasound is discussed again later in this chapter.

Progress of pregnancy

For most women, once pregnancy is confirmed, everything proceeds smoothly. There may be a little nausea in the early morning, due to the body having to adjust to new high levels of hormones, but this usually passes off after the first few weeks, as does frequency of urination which is only due to the kidneys functioning particularly efficiently.

A woman's whole body has to adapt to the new demands being made on it, and it should really be exciting and rewarding to feel this happening. Nature has devised things so that the baby has first call and priority. This only becomes a crucial factor where a mother is under-nourished, but it does mean a balanced diet is important. As the growing foetus increases its demands for oxygen, food and efficient waste-disposal, the mother usually finds herself becoming more placid and conserving energy, so that fat starts to be deposited on breasts, hips and thighs.

This slowing down process is natural and necessary, but it

has the one disadvantage of also affecting the gut, so that the stomach may empty more slowly and there may sometimes be a problem with constipation. Diet can usually overcome this, and high bulk, low energy foods such as bran are very important and helpful, but in any case a safe remedy can always be prescribed. It's important *not* to go in for purgatives or indeed any sort of self-medication during pregnancy. The more drugs can be avoided the better, and that goes for smoking too. It has been proved beyond doubt that smoking will reduce the birth weight and can adversely affect foetal breathing and health both in the short and longer term, as well as increasing the risk of miscarriage.

A Cardiff study showed twice as many babies born to mothers who smoked were badly underweight, and twice as many had congenital heart disease. There were also more with cleft palates and hare lips. In the longer term, a survey in this country of some 17 000 children followed from birth showed that at the age of eleven those whose mothers had smoked were between five and seven months behind in mental ability compared to children of non-smokers.

You would think the evidence from all sides was now strong enough to dissuade expectant mothers from smoking. They normally have a highly protective approach to their babies even before they are born. Yet the 1970 Cardiff study showed 15 per cent of pregnant women smoking more than twenty cigarettes a day compared to only 4 per cent back in 1964.

Pregnancy certainly does not demand sacrifice of all pleasures. Moderate exercise and gentle intercourse are both good, and for many couples it can be a time of special sexual pleasure with no contraceptive measures needed.

While alcohol in moderation does no harm, there is evidence of increasing numbers of seriously deformed babies or mentally retarded babies born to mothers who drink heavily. Studies in both the USA and Germany have shown adverse effects on birthweight, growth and head circumference. The death rate among babies born to alcoholics was more than eight times that of babies born to other mothers.

Fortunately, both excessive smoking and compulsive drinking are special problems confined to the few, and it's not easy for the rest of us to understand the difficulty of kicking such addictions. But if ever there was a time to try, and a good reason to do so, it's when a woman is pregnant.

For most women with no such problems, pregnancy is a happy and contented time, with exciting preparations to make, plenty to think about and plan, and constant new physical experiences to savour.

Breast changes

A lot of women experience breast discomfort just prior to a menstrual period and in pregnancy a similar feeling occurs and persists with the breasts becoming fuller, firmer and slightly tender. As pregnancy advances the nipples become larger and darker and small protuberances may appear around them, due to the enlargement of tiny milk glands and ducts. This can lead to throbbing or tingling sensations, but for the women anxious to breast-feed, these will be a welcome sign that her own personal dairy is being set up.

Quickening

This is the old word for the first faint movements of the baby usually felt at about eighteen to twenty weeks of pregnancy. It's a strange and exciting feeling, and quickening is an odd term to use for it, but it derives from the old Biblical phrase, 'the quick and the dead', because it used to be thought that this was the moment at which the baby became alive.

Movement becomes strong and more frequent as the baby grows and exercises inside the safe insulated environment of the womb. Some babies are more active than others, and with some there can be long periods without movement which most certainly does *not* mean the baby is dead. If a woman becomes really worried, however, after an unusually long time with no movement at all, she should reassure herself by seeing her doctor. He will listen for the foetal heart and even allow the mother to hear it herself. That is a great moment. As mentioned, the ultrasound machine can also be used if there is any problem in locating the baby's heartbeat.

E

Heart-rate changes

The needs of the growing baby demand a 40 per cent increase in the volume of the mother's blood and its more rapid circulation. This forces the heart to beast faster and some women complain of palpitations. All it means is that the blood is being pumped more rapidly to carry the vital oxygen and nutrients which cross the placenta to reach the baby.

As well as nutrients and drugs, the placenta also allows passage of what are called antibodies. These are substances formed by our bodies specifically to attack and destroy harmful invading germs. Antibodies made by the mother during her life remain present in her own blood, and can cross the placenta to confer some protection on the baby, until it can begin to manufacture its own antibodies quite soon after birth.

It's this normally protective system that was found to underlie the mysterious problem of babies born so badly jaundiced that they usually died, before the reason became fully understood and treatment developed.

The Rhesus factor

That reason was found to be a special antigen, which is the name given to a substance which stimulates formation of an antibody to counteract it. This particular antigen became known as the Rhesus antigen or Rhesus factor, because during experiments to discover it, a serum was prepared from the red cells of Rhesus monkeys, all of whom were found to possess this particular antigen.

If all humans also possessed the Rhesus factor there would be no problem. But roughly 15 per cent of Caucasians lack it and are known as Rhesus negative. The 85 per cent who have it are known as Rhesus positive.

If it was only Rhesus positive women and Rhesus positive men who were attracted to each other, there would be no problem. But human beings do not fall in love or mate to order according to blood groups and factors. So by the law of averages about 10 per cent of conceptions will involve a Rhesus negative of one sex and a Rhesus positive from the other.

With a first baby this does not usually matter. Even if the mother is Rhesus negative and the baby proves to have inherited

Rhesus positive blood from the father, only very small amounts will have seeped through to the placenta during the pregnancy to enter the mother's blood stream. This small amount is usually successfully destroyed by the mother's antibodies.

But at delivery of this first baby, far larger amounts of the baby's blood may get into the mother's blood stream, often too great to allow the Rhesus factor to be destroyed, so the mother's immune system goes into action manufacturing vast regiments of antibodies which will remain there on the alert, ready to attack any Rhesus positive cells which should enter her body at a later date.

That later date may well be during a second pregnancy if that baby is also Rhesus positive. So a second time round the dangerous mechanism is already triggered and, as the pregnancy progresses, the mother's antibodies seek out and attack the red blood cells of her own baby to destroy the alien Rhesus positive cells. As this happens, the baby becomes more and more anaemic, and in the past it usually died.

But once again we are so lucky today that medicine has come to the rescue and such tragedies can now usually be avoided. Initially, tests are done to establish whether an expectant mother is Rhesus negative. If she is, and if her husband proves to be Rhesus positive, the next step is to see if her blood already contains antibodies. If so, then doctors know there may be risk to the baby if it has Rhesus positive blood. In the past, transfusions were given in these cases to keep them alive, if necessary even while the baby was still in the womb.

But now treatment is available which virtually eliminates the whole problem. Its success depends on treating any Rhesus negative women *before* her body has been stimulated to produce the antibodies which attack Rhesus positive blood. So all women are tested at *first* pregnancy. If they are Rhesus negatige, a painless injection is given any time up to 72 hours after the birth of a Rhesus positive baby. This destroys any Rhesus positive cells from the baby which may have penetrated her blood stream, making it unnecessary for her own body to produce the antibodies which would endanger future pregnancies.

If it all sounds a bit confusing, the main thing to remember is that it works, and so do even more recently developed methods of vaccinating against German measles.

The German measles danger

German measles (also called rubella) is caused by a virus which has a particularly nasty preference for newly forming tissue. Because of this, if a woman contracts German measles before the tenth week of pregnancy, the virus tends to home in on the heart, ears or skull of the foetus, all of which are forming at that time.

As a result the baby's heart may be damaged, hearing impaired or eyes badly affected, while the skull may fail to expand and allow proper brain development. These horrible complications are known to affect over half of all babies whose mothers catch German measles during this vital period of early pregnancy. So to prevent the tragedy of deformed babies being born, all that could be done in the past was to terminate pregnancy in women who had contracted German measles any time during the first twelve weeks of pregnancy.

Again a simpler and more humane answer has now been found. A simple test can indicate now if a woman has ever had German measles. Many of us have it as children without ever knowing, and once we have had it there is *no* possibility of ever having it again so no risk during pregnancy. But if the test shows a woman has *not* had the disease, then a mild attack can now be provoked by a special vaccine and this will safeguard her in exactly the same way against any further infection. Until this vital injection has had time to take effect, for about two months, it is important for really safe forms of birth control to be used if intercourse is taking place. German measles vaccine is now routinely offered to all girls between the ages of eleven and fourteen and they are well advised to accept.

Genetic counselling

You may have wondered how doctors could tell if a baby in the womb was Rhesus positive, and the answer to this and many other questions about the unborn baby lies in a process called amniocentesis.

This is a method, only developed in recent years, which allows the amniotic fluid surrounding the baby to be sampled. Again it is a quite painless procedure using a local anaesthetic and then inserting a hollow needle very carefully through the mother's abdomen. A small amount of amniotic fluid is drawn up and from this cells from the actual foetus can be separated out.

Examined chemically and under a microscope, these can now provide invaluable information about the baby, revealing the presence or absence of genetic disorders which at one time could only be guessed at.

In the past what was termed genetic counselling was very much a question of mathematics, of calculating the odds of some hereditary defect or disease being passed on. Where both parents *carry* the same defective genes, for example, the risk of any children inheriting an increased risk of the disease was estimated at one in four. If both parents actually suffered from the disease, the odds were known to be even worse.

But now, by using amniocentesis, the agony of fear and doubt can be resolved. Joe Jordan, consultant gynaecologist, explained to me the situation.

We can do these tests as early as sixteen weeks after conception, but we only do them where there is real reason, where a baby may suffer from spina bifida for instance.

Some one per cent of babies abort after amniocentesis, so we do not use it lightly. It's very sad that this means a few normal babies are lost, but others would have died anyway from abnormalities and so on balance it means a great deal of suffering is saved. If the pregnancy proves normal, then the terrible anxiety is removed and it can go ahead with the parents happy and confident. If we do find serious abnormality, then the parents are told and they almost invariably ask for termination rather than bring a seriously affected baby into the world.

For example, one defective gene allows poisons to build up, causing convulsions and brain damage and again, by knowing in advance, it can often be countered by putting babies on a special diet.

In women in premature labour, amniocentesis can determine beforehand if the baby will have blocked lungs and breathing difficulties, and labour can be delayed until delivery is safe.

At King's College Hospital and at University College Hospital in London, another even more delicate pre-natal diagnosis is being used in certain special cases.

Stuart Campbell, professor of obstetrics at King's College explained this method, called fetoscopy.

> We also insert a hollow needle, but this has a light source so that we can actually look down it and see the foetus. It is a very skilled technique [he warned] as we need to locate blood vessels in the placenta and then insert another narrower needle, through which we draw out a little blood which comes only from the unborn baby. From this we can detect the sort of gene defects which produce blood abnormalities such as sickle-cell anaemia.

Ten per cent of black people carry this defective gene, and another faulty gene, producing a different form of anaemia, is carried by 15 per cent of the Mediterranean races. Professor Campbell says:

> We have set up our special units here to cater for the large West Indian and Cypriot population. It's a service which should be available, particularly for mothers who have already had the tragic experience of bearing one affected child. We also hope to train doctors from Africa and the Mediterranean countries, so that they can go back and carry out the services among their own people where they are so badly needed.

Mongolism

This is another chromosome defect disease which amniocentesis can check on. But something just as simple as good family planning is also helping tremendously to reduce this problem. The fault occurs when one certain chromosome is present *three* times instead of the correct twice in every cell. It has been known for a long time that this happens more often during the development of the eggs of older women. The risk of a mongol baby is only one in 1000 for mothers under the age of twenty-five but rises to one in forty for mothers over forty, and an incredible one in eight for mothers over forty-five.[26]

Mr Jordan told me, 'I believe all expectant mothers over 35, and certainly those over 40, should have a pre-natal check done by amniocentesis. It can prevent so many tragedies.'

This is obviously good advice in view of the high risk rate for older women. Fortunately, thanks to better contraception, fewer older women now get pregnant. In Japan, family planning alone has reduced mongol babies by between 20 and 40 per cent; in Germany and in this country, even by 1964, mongol-ism had been reduced by 25 per cent. With better education about the increased risk, and with contraception now free, the figures for the U K should soon be even lower.

Another very helpful development is a preliminary blood test which can indicate whether a baby is likely to be at risk from spina bifida. If so, then of course amniocentesis must be the next step, but it means it can be avoided in cases where the result of the blood test is negative.

Miscarriages

For a woman happy in her pregnancy and badly wanting a baby, even early miscarriages must seem a tragedy. But in fact there is a different way of looking at it in the light of modern medical knowledge. We now know that nature itself exercises a fairly ruthless system of quality control, and one in three of conceptions which spontaneously miscarry early on are found to have genetic abnormalities. Other defective fertilized eggs are lost because they are unable even to attach themselves to the wall of the womb for implantation and development. At St Bartholomew's hospital in London, Dr Yehudi Gordon, researching in this field, told me, 'Our work suggests perhaps as many as 80 per cent of fertilized eggs fail to implant. The woman just has a late period or a heavier bleed and never realises she was pregnant.'

The usual estimated figure for spontaneous abortion which is the correct medical term for 'miscarriage' is one in seven. Only one third may have genetic defects but three-quarters of them are abnormal in some way, so the loss must not be looked upon entirely as a tragedy. It is a disappointment but there will be other pregnancies, less precarious and promising a healthier baby.

The first sign of impending or threatened abortion is usually bleeding. This may start as irregular spotting followed later by a moderate discharge resembling a period. In other cases the bleeding may be heavy right from the start and be accompanied by cramping pains. Although it's natural to be worried and a doctor should always be consulted at once, it's reassuring to know that 80 per cent of such threatened abortions do settle down and pregnancy continues to a normal delivery and a normal baby.

The usual treatment is bed rest for a few days, with intercourse to be avoided for a couple of weeks. If this does not result in the bleeding stopping, the chances are that the miscarriage is inevitable. It is also likely that there is good reason for it and so a philosophical acceptance is the best way, though that is no doubt easier said than done.

But just as light falls, blows on the tummy or even emotional shock are now known not really to threaten a healthy wellfounded pregnancy, so also will nothing really preserve an unhealthy and precarious one.

There are women, however, who habitually abort and then the position is rather different. In these cases blood or urine tests may be done to check on levels of progesterone, the hormone which particularly preserves pregnancy. If levels are low, pure progesterone may be given in the form of injections or dydrogesterone given by mouth. This is the retroprogesterone, so similar in structure to pure progesterone, and already mentioned in association with pre-menstrual tension for which it is also used.

One increasingly common reason for miscarriages these days is a weakness of the neck of the womb, often the result of repeated abortions where the cervix has been dilated. A simple stitch round the cervix and pulled tight to keep it closed can save about three-quarters of the babies who might otherwise be lost for this reason.

Sometimes bleeding in early pregnancy may only prove to be what is called implantation bleeding as the egg burrows its way in. Sometimes it may be a sign of an ectopic pregnancy as already mentioned. Either way it must be reported and investigated.

Bleeding late on in pregnancy is usually the result of a portion of the placenta becoming separated from its bed in the wall of the womb. That invaluable ultrasound machine can usually establish this, and whether the baby is far enough advanced to survive. If so, about four patients in ten go on to normal delivery and the other six may well have a Caesarean, which is explained later in this chapter.

Toxaemia in pregnancy

This is the name most often used (but totally inappropriate) for swelling of fingers, face or legs, with a rise in blood pressure and appearance of protein in the urine, which can occur usually late in pregnancy. The reason for it is not understood but it affects about 12 per cent of first pregnancies and 6 per cent of later ones. There is really no connection with toxins or poisons, and the correct name is pre-eclampsia.

Eclampsia itself is what the condition may progress to if neglected, and this is serious with possible convulsions and a considerable threat to the baby.

Although most of the complications described here are rare, the point of mentioning them is to emphasize that for the sake of the baby and herself, an expectant mother should attend for regular antenatal visits, so that blood pressure is checked, weight gain noted, urine examined and any possible troubles anticipated and dealt with. 'Better safe than sorry' is good advice at any time and never more so than during pregnancy when you are responsible for two lives.

Pregnancy toxaemia may be dealt with by simply restricting the diet, particularly the amount of salt used, taking diuretic tablets to get rid of excess water and by increased rest at home. If this is not fully effective than it may be a question of admission to hospital.

Even in a factual book like this it is tempting at some point to indulge in the luxury of a personal anecdote. My own perfectly healthy first pregnancy suddenly flared at eight months into a raging toxaemia. It was summer and as always at that time of year I was very sun-tanned, so maybe that had helped disguise any symptoms under a veneer of well-being. Fortunately a perceptive physiotherapist friend noticed my puffy fingers plus a generally slightly bloated look under the tan and a quick check by my doctor showed soaring blood pressure. Within an hour I found myself swept off to Birmingham Maternity Hospital complete with my bag, fortunately already packed and ready.

Although I appreciated the sound medical reasons for putting me into a quiet small ward, I was to find the psychological reasoning a bit shaky. I soon discovered that every one of the eight or nine women in that side ward had already lost their babies. It was not a very encouraging start.

In retrospect I think it was just as bad for them, but they were marvellous and cheered me on through the first stages of labour as I strived to keep up my relaxation breathing. A surgical induction had been done to try and save the baby and I was lucky – a perfect baby girl, three weeks premature and only weighing 5½ lbs but no real problems.

I was tactfully moved after the birth into the normal large public ward but not allowed to stir a foot out of bed as the blood pressure was still dangerously high. I still remember vividly feeling a terrible fraud, lying there brown as a berry and waited on hand and foot by pale fragile looking fellow-patients. I got such a complex about it, as they carried bowls for me to wash in and generally looked after me, that I printed a large notice, WORSE THAN SHE LOOKS, and hung it on the end of the bed.

Once your baby is safely born the public ward of a Maternity Hospital is tremendous fun and I was horrified when Sister decided to move me to a quiet private ward, as I was obviously enjoying myself far too much and the blood pressure was staying obstinately up. In case anyone is interested in the comparison, the private ward was much less fun and the food exactly the same.

The decision as to where you are going to have your baby is an important one. Quite frankly for any *first* baby there is no really sensible option other than the nearest and/or best hospital with a specialist maternity department.

I do understand very well the recent outcry against the battery-hen, conveyor-belt system which in some areas was allowed to squeeze the humanity out of this most human and personal of experiences. But lessons have been learned and a real effort is being made now to reverse the trend and get back to childbirth as a shared experience for the parents. Babies are born into families not just into labour wards or delivery rooms. Most hospitals now encourage the father to be present if he wishes. Most of the consultants I have talked to about the situation are very conscious of the need to make the hospital experience congenial, less impersonal, less daunting and give the first-time mother reassurance and company during labour.

Too much emphasis has undoubtedly been put in some hospitals on technical advances and too little on old-fashioned informality and fellow-feeling.

Today the move is toward shorter hospital stays. If all goes well and the mother has got adequate arrangements at home and wants to go back, often forty-eight hours is all she needs to spend in hospital. The chances are all will go smoothly as it does for four out of five births. But it is not possible to predict accurately which is the one which may present problems.

A woman gives up nine months of her life to gestating the baby in her womb and another eighteen years legally to its care – usually she gives a whole life-time of love. So, really it's strange that she should take any risk or refuse to give those vital 48 hours which can perhaps make so much difference to giving the baby a good start. If for any reason it is born in a distressed condition, it needs to have incubators and all the latest medical aids on hand. My own choice would be hospital every time and home as soon as possible. For some women with other small demanding children and exhausting lives, it might even be the best chance ever for a rest and a bit of 'spoiling'.

There is a better case if all has gone well with a first baby for the second and even the third to be born at home, if a woman feels strongly and if there is good care available. After the third baby, even according to doctors who favour home confinement for numbers two and three, all further births should once again be in hospital.

It is not possible to generalize on this subject. So much depends on the situation in your area, in your home, in the community nursing care available and your own doctor's attitude.

Monitoring in pregnancy and labour

Modern means of monitoring growth and progress of the baby both during pregnancy and during labour are together helping to produce healthier babies, reduce the duration and trauma of labour and reducing infant and maternal mortality.

One of the most common reasons in the past for babies being born very weak and sometimes even dead was undetected 'placental deficiency'. That means the placenta had aged prematurely and was no longer able to do its iob and keep the baby in the womb supplied with sufficient oxygen. One reason for this can be high blood pressure in the mother and another, as mentioned earlier, can be cigarette-smoking during pregnancy.

There can obviously be many other reasons too but in what is called the high risk mother, the function of the placenta can be simply checked by taking twenty-four-hour urine collections from the mother twice a week. From these the levels of oestriol are measured, an oestrogen produced both by the placenta and the unborn baby's adrenal gland. Any fall in oestriol indicates the need for further careful follow-up monitoring and here ultrasound comes into action. As we have already seen this works like wartime sonar, but not to detect hostile submarines moving through the wide waters of the sea, but to follow the progress of one small baby in its own limited watery environment inside the mother.

The special use of ultrasound can be combined with cardiotocography which involves electrodes being attached to the mother's abdomen, just stuck to the surface skin. These focus the ultrasound waves in the direction of the foetal chest and pick up the baby's heart rate, which is then shown on a screen as a tracing. Any severe lack of oxygen is reflected by irregular foetal heart rate and in late pregnancy this, plus decreased foetal movement which the ultrasound will also reveal, may well indicate that it is safer to induce premature labour than leave the baby in a failing placenta.

Induction

A certain amount of misunderstanding about inductions and some misrepresentation in the media have led some women to resist or refuse to be induced, even when doctors advise it as necessary to help the baby. Usually a careful explanation will overcome this fear, but the area of misunderstanding, which is often largely responsible for such reluctance, is publicity about the increase in the number of Caesarean births following induction of labour. There is a higher incidence, but this is due to the complications of pregnancy which made the induction necessary, *not* because of the induction technique itself. Inductions are certainly not done without good reason or purely for the convenience of doctors and staff, though they may sometimes be justified to try and ensure a baby is born when anaesthetic and laboratory facilities are easily available during daytime hours.

Placental failure, toxaemia, haemorrhage or pregnancy prolonged to more than forty-two weeks are all good reasons for induction. The usual method is simply for the bag of water to be cut with a small instrument. The waters run out through cervix and vagina and within a short time labour usually starts. The process is painless though with feet up in stirrups hardly dignified, as I found myself when this same method was used years ago to induce my daughter into the world when she was threatened by my high blood pressure and toxaemia. Frankly most women soon come to terms with a few indignities in the cause of medical care and safety for themselves and their babies. Giving birth is not an elegant business – exciting, amazing, incredible, shattering, fantastic – almost any of these adjectives might apply but dignity has little to do with the irresistible primitive process of producing new life. When nature takes over there is nothing exactly dignified about it, except perhaps for the way most women cope with it and come up smiling at the end when their baby is placed in their arms.

The real key to the correct use of induction, now recognized by the medical profession, is careful monitoring with use of ultrasound to ensure the baby is mature and able to survive. Occasionally, by relying on dates of the last period and ordinary examination, babies were induced too soon; dates had been miscalculated and they were sometimes at risk. It can be a difficult decision because, if not induced, they can be at even higher risk. Regular ultrasound monitoring can enable the right judgement to be made, by confirming the correct dates and detecting any decreased rate of growth of the unborn baby.

Sometimes labour is started by using an oxytocin drip. This drug, which stimulates the uterus to contract, is simply run at a controlled rate into an arm vein and this method is also used, if necessary, to accelerate labour after it has started spontaneously but is rather too slow.

John Studd, consultant gynaecologist at King's College Hospital, who has contributed a great deal to the safety of labour for women in this country, told me:

These days we can avoid the hazards of placental failure or prolonged labour. In the past, after thirty-six hours or more of distressing labour, it was common for a Caesarean section to be performed
on an exhausted mother, who subsequently retained a scar on her
uterus and on her memory, resolving never to become pregnant
again. If necessary today, labour can be safely induced and, equally
important, labour occurring spontaneously, which is recognized as
progressing at a slower rate than normal, can be accelerated. No
woman today should be in labour for more than twelve hours.

If the key to the correct medical decision about induction
lies with ultrasound, the key to whether acceleration of labour
is required lies with something called a partogram.

This is a means of recording the progress of labour on a
graph so that any variation from the normal rate can be
picked up at once. It was designed originally by Professor Hugh
Philpott, who first used it out in Rhodesia. In areas with poor
social services and poor transport facilities, partograms and the
accurate indication they gave of where acceleration of labour
was needed, reduced still-births by a dramatic 75 per cent.

John Studd, who was working in Africa at the time, brought
the idea back and introduced partograms to this country,
working out the graph shapes and slopes of normal progression
of labour for *our* population, so that the necessary comparisons
could be made, and patients identified who needed help to
speed things up to avoid distress or danger to themselves and
their babies.[27]

John Studd emphasized, 'The use of the partogram is just as
important in indicating the patient who does *not* need oxytocin
drip and acceleration of labour. Our object is never to speed up
normally progressing labour, but only to ensure that labour is
not allowed to become dangerously prolonged through our
neglect.'

While partograms display the progress of labour, another
print-out is frequently used to monitor the foetal heart-rate
during the birth. A small electrode is placed on the baby's
scalp as it becomes accessible in its descent down the birth
canal. If what are called 'dips' in the print-out suggest further
checks may be needed, blood can be taken quite easily and
safely from the baby's scalp. This sounds horrific but it is quite
simple and done under direct vision through the vagina. Just

a tiny stab incision is made and a drop of blood sucked up a capillary tube. The degree of acidosis in this blood sample will accurately reflect any oxygen deficiency and indicate if there is sufficient foetal distress to require forceps to bring the baby or, if the cervix is not fully dilated, perhaps delivery by Caesarean section.

Forceps delivery

Using instruments to fetch the baby used to be thought of by the woman as a serious and dreaded business. Today the skill of the doctors and the tremendous improvement in the instruments used make forceps deliveries safe and nothing to fear. In fact, a sort of flat cap or cup pushed against the head of the baby is often used in conjunction with a vacuum suction effect, just helping the baby down and with this method there is even less risk of damage to the mother's tissues.

Episiotomy

Occasionally a deliberate small cut is made in the perineum (the pelvic floor) if the doctor feels it will aid delivery and this is called an episiotomy. It should *not* be used routinely, but if it is necessary and is skilfully stitched up, there is only slight discomfort for a day or two.

Caesarean section

This has been referred to once or twice already in this book and most women know what it means. The word comes from the Latin *caedere*, to cut, and if for any reason the baby cannot be born through the birth canal, or the length of labour makes it advisable to revert to Caesarean section, then the mother is just given a general anaesthetic and an incision is made in the lower part of the abdominal wall. The baby is simply lifted out through this incision, which is then closed with stitches. In some ways Caesarean section could be considered the easy way to have a baby, because the mother just wakes up to find it is all over and probably to hear her baby crying and feel it placed in her arms.

The old adage, 'once a Caesarean, always a Caesarean', certainly does not apply these days, and many women have further babies by normal delivery. Only about 6 per cent of babies are delivered by Caesarean in this country and about double that percentage in America.

Relief of pain in labour

Reactions to labour contractions vary enormously. Some women can cope well throughout, with no sedatives or analgesics, but others are glad of help and today will get it. For the nervous woman sedatives can help a great deal, and sometimes these are given by injection into the muscle when labour is under way to give a nice relaxed feeling.

Toward the end of the first stage of labour and in the second stage, the mother may want further help to reduce pain or discomfort. Pethidine given by injection into the muscle, usually in the thigh, dulls pain very quickly and lasts for two to five hours so that more than one injection may be given. Over many years' use now, it has proved safe and effective.

Two anaesthetic mixtures are also used which the mother controls herself, by putting a mask to her face and breathing deeply during contractions. One mixture consists of nitrous oxide and oxygen and is perhaps most commonly used. The other is called Trilene and is a sweet-smelling blue liquid which vaporizes when air is passed over it. The Trilene is placed in the inhaler and as the mother breathes in air it passes over the Trilene and the vapour from it dulls the pain.

Epidural anaesthesia

This is the most effective of all methods of pain relief and is entirely safe in skilled hands. It works by blocking the passage of messages from the nerves which relay the sensation of pain involved in contractions. This is why it's often called 'an epidural block'. The anaesthetist inserts a thin needle through the muscles of the mother's back getting the tip to lie in just the right place. He then pushes a very fine polythene tube through the needle which is then withdrawn, leaving the tube still in position. Down this tube local anaesthetic can be fed as needed, topping up when the effect begins to wear off, so that pain is relieved but the patient is fully conscious and able to co-operate.

The one snag with this method, which has led to some controversy, is that during the final phase of labour when the mother is required to push or 'bear down' to help the baby's final emergence, she is not able to register precisely the moment and so sometimes this leads to a higher incidence of forceps deliveries.

Pudendal block

This is a very effective means of anaesthetizing the birth outlet for the final phase of labour, when the baby's head begins to stretch the tissues around the vulva to give what women often describe as a 'bursting feeling'. It may be used at this stage to obliterate pain in normal deliveries but even more often for forceps or suction extraction.

Instead of the rather more tricky spinal injection the pudendal block simply consists of injection of local anaesthetic by a long fine needle passed through the skin beside the vagina; the tip is guided by the doctor's finger to the spiny process of the pelvis around which are the pudendal nerves, which transmit sensation from the vaginal area. Blocking these nerves on each side relieves the mother of unnecessary pain as instruments are inserted or as the outlet is stretched during the birth.

So there are now many ways and many new techniques being used to make having a baby easier and safer. Modern medicine aims to leave the woman as healthy or even more healthy at the end of pregnancy and childbirth than at the start, and to achieve a live and undamaged baby for her.

At one time there was a bit of a cult about natural childbirth and of course it's a splendid theory and a splendid achievement if all goes to plan. But so often nature is only a good doctor or good midwife in terms of survival of the species – that is what nature is all about – it cares little for the individual or individual suffering or safety. In fact nature and evolution are designed to allow survival of the fittest. Left to nature some babies and some mothers will die, but enough will survive to keep the human race going – that is nature's only concern.

So we are fortunate to live in an age when help can be given when needed and when the value of every human being is recognized. But I believe we are also fortunate to be able to assess in advance the chances for 'quality of life', and with proper counselling to give parents the chance of termination if that quality will not be there, and if a badly damaged baby destined for a lifetime of suffering is likely to be born.

Breast-feeding

It is not really within the scope of this book to look at baby and child-care, but the modern recognition of the great value of breast-feeding seems to me to be worth emphasizing.

With the advent of artificial baby foods, which can be bought over the counter, with greater affluence, less help in the home, and perhaps a more sophisticated approach to living, breast-feeding went out of fashion for a long time. One survey in Cardiff, only a few years ago, showed by the seventh day after birth only a third of mothers were giving breast milk, and that figure continued to decline in succeeding weeks.

Yet the advantages of breast-feeding are very real, very immediate, and probably even last into adult life. Human breast milk is sterile, balanced and appropriate to the human baby. Cow's milk in contrast is appropriate to calves and contains protein foreign to the human and difficult to digest. Human milk contains more lactose (milk sugar) than cow's milk, more vitamins and more minerals, and it is certainly more hygienic. As one doctor put it to me, 'The cat can't get at it and it comes in such cute containers.'

Certainly the formula milks made for bottle-feeding are modified from cow's milk to make them as much like human milk as possible, but there is no way in which they can mimic the subtle substances in human breast milk which confer immunity and protection on the young baby, nor can the bottle forge quite the same bond as a warm soft breast.

The mother who can manage to feed her baby, if possible just for the first three months, gives it not only the best sort of milk in the best sort of container, designed for built-in hygiene and convenience. Even more importantly, she gives it her own resistance to disease, until the baby is big enough to have had the chance to begin to build up its own immunity.

In the past, the rigid routine of hospitals, with babies kept in separate nurseries and brought to the mothers only at fixed hours, often led to difficulties in milk production because of restricted contact and suckling. This led in turn to supplementary feeds with formula milk, a sense of failure and frustration on the mother's part, and probably emotional upset which could further suppress milk production. Often there was no one in the busy hospital (where the value of breast-feeding was not appreciated anyway) to give the help and encouragement which might be needed to get breast-feeding established for a new mother and baby. Not all babies automatically take to the nipple and start suckling – some babies are lazy, some nipples inverted – and without expert help it was often easier just to give up and resort to the feeding bottle, however much a woman might originally have hoped to breast-feed.

Happily things have changed. The value of breast-feeding is not only recognized now on medical grounds but also on psychological grounds, as the importance of the early bond formed between mother and baby and the role of breast-feeding, contact and cuddling in this bond forming is ackknowledged.

Another major factor in the swing toward breast-feeding has been recent work showing the dangers of over-feeding with bottle-fed babies. With breast-feeding it's almost impossible to over-feed, but it is very tempting with bottle-feeding to just add that extra scoop of milk powder and this leads to more fat in the fat cells and to more fat cells than normal, producing not merely fat babies, but unfortunately fat adolescents and fat adults. There is evidence that this can lead in the longer term to increased heart-disease and so breast-feeding a baby may well protect the adult against what is still the greatest killer.

What is called demand feeding has considerable medical support today, and this is really just the natural way of feeding the baby when it is hungry as mothers have always done before down the ages. It was really only in this century, due largely to hospital routine, that the system emerged of regular three- or four-hourly feeds, and disciplined feeding and *not* picking up the crying baby became part of modern baby-law.

Today, as we have already seen, a better balance is being struck between science and nature and between modern technology and ancient instinct. Enlightened hospitals are already recognizing the value of allowing mother and baby to be much more together, so that the young mother learns to recognize and distinguish between the different cries of hunger, boredom and discomfort. Even tiny babies get bored and with the baby beside her the mother can stimulate, comfort, cuddle or change nappies as needed, but above all she can feed the baby when it's hungry, not just when nurse brings it in for a scheduled feed, sometimes even having to wake it out of peaceful sleep in order to stick to the timetable.

Anyone watching a baby breast-feeding can be left in no doubt of the comfort and security it gains and the extra dimension of sensual satisfaction the breast gives. For most women too it is rewarding and relaxing. The old idea that breast-feeding will spoil the figure has been proved quite untrue and nor will it cause the breasts to sag, providing during the last weeks of pregnancy a well-fitting brassiere has been worn day and night and this is continued during the breast-feeding period.

The breast-feeding mother does not have to eat vast quantities of food, and in fact the stores of fat she has built up during pregnancy are there to serve this very period and purpose – that is why they were laid down and they will be used up in the breast-feeding process. Nor is breast-feeding going to tire the mother out, as so often old-wives' tales would have it. With the good balanced diet available to most of us in the West today, breast-feeding is possible for most women who want to do it and is quite likely to be less exhausting than all the business of sterilizing and preparing bottle feeds. Of course caring for any small baby, especially the first one when you are inexperienced, can be tiring, and with breast-feeding or bottle-feeding, you are still going to benefit from all the rest and relaxation you can manage to get.

Derek Llewellyn-Jones's superb book, *Everywoman*, of which details are given at the back, makes a strong case for breast-feeding and gives excellent tips on techniques. His message is 'breast-feeding is best-feeding', but it still has to be recognized that it is not always possible. Some women, to their bitter disappointment, find for various reasons they cannot do it or cannot keep it up. Others quite genuinely find it repellent, an attitude which can stem from their own upbringing perhaps rooted in the idea that exposure of the breast is immodest. Others resent the interference breast-feeding may impose on social life, and still others may have urgent economic reasons for needing to get back to work.

So finally it should be said that the mother who cannot breast-feed for either medical or psychological reasons must not feel she has failed her baby or failed as a mother. There are fine products available, and all she must do is be sure that she uses them wisely and correctly and makes a special point of plenty of cuddling between feeds to establish the same warm bond and sense of closeness and security all babies need. Like so much else in life, the choice should be an individual one. Doctors and even perhaps medical journalists like me can recommend and point out the pros and cons, but each individual woman must make her own decision in the light of her own circumstances and feelings. The exception to this freedom of choice seems to me to be in the selfish indulgence of anything positively harmful to the baby such as smoking.

10. Female disorders

In considering the main health problems and disorders that particularly affect women and raise all sorts of fears and anxiety, at the very top of the list must obviously come female forms of cancer.

Until recently the very word was one which many people could not even bring themselves to utter. 'Has she got you-know-what?' they would mouth, or, 'Is it *it*?' and deep down inside everyone of us even now probably lurks the fear whenever strange symptoms occur that it may be the dreaded disease.

In fact, of course, cancer is not in itself a disease – the term really covers a whole group of conditions which have the one thing in common, namely, something has gone wrong with the normal controlled process of cell division so that cells have gone wild and grow where they shouldn't.

Massive research is going on round the world with vast amounts of money being spent to try and find out why this happens, to prevent it, reverse it and cure it. The answer will almost certainly be found at the cell level and meanwhile new methods are reducing mortality in some areas of cancer and better screening methods, more widely available, are aiding early diagnosis, which is the real key to the problem.

All this is helping to bring the subject into the open and destroying the old myths. Cancer is wrongly rated as the disease that kills most people and as being incurable. In fact heart disease is still the great killer and cancer caught early is usually curable.

But early diagnosis demands publicity, vigilance and co-operation, and in no area is this more important that in the commonest of all cancers in women, breast cancer.

Breast cancer

About five in every 100 women will develop breast cancer at some time. It is a frightening figure and a hard fact to face. But there is another fact. While breast cancer in its late stages is usually incurable, in its early stages there is a 90 per cent cure success rate. But early means just that, and every woman should supplement regular annual or biannual checks with her doctor or family planning clinic by doing a regular monthly breast examination herself, preferably seven days after starting each menstrual period. After the menopause, when menstruation has finished and when in fact the risk of breast cancer increases, it is even more important to carry out the check regularly each month. This should become a routine five-minute job for every woman over the age of thirty-five for the rest of her life.

Excellent illustrated leaflets can be obtained from family planning clinics or from doctors' surgeries, and a very good booklet is also available from the Health Council and is listed at the back. Meanwhile here is one recommended way of doing your own check-up.

First stand or sit in front of a mirror and just look for any changes in breast size or shape, also for any puckering or dimpling of the skin. Raise your hands above your head and observe the breasts again from that position. Finally gently squeeze the nipples and look to see if there is any discharge or any particular change in them. Remember that not all nipple discharges are sinister. A yellowish secretion is common in women who have had children, incompleted pregnancies or who are on the Pill. But all unusual findings should be reported just to be on the safe side.

Next lie down with a pillow or bath-towel under the left shoulder and the left hand under the head. With fingers of the right hand feel carefully for any lumps or thickening. To do this the fingers should be held flat and pressed gently but firmly with a small circular motion. Work methodically first feeling the inner-upper portion of the breast, moving from the breastbone outward toward the nipple and then repeating this for the inner-lower part. Also feel round the nipple and note any sudden inversion.

The next stage is to bring the left arm down to your side. Still using flat finger tips feel under the armpits, then with the same gentle pressure feel the upper-outer quarter of the breast from the nipple line to where your arm is resting.

Finally check the lower-outer section, this time working from the outer part in toward the nipple. Then repeat the whole procedure for the right breast.

The old idea that a blow on the breast can precipitate cancer is perhaps worth demolishing at this stage. A blow can sometimes produce a lump, due to destruction of fat cells, and this may have to be removed to distinguish it from a malignancy. The point is that such an accident can often lead to a medical consultation, and this can sometimes reveal existing though *un*related trouble, which may obviously help to perpetuate and build the myth.

Breast cancer is not common in younger women. In the teens and twenties, a lump usually proves to be what is rather charmingly called a 'breast mouse', a harmless tumour given its name because it can be felt moving or running under the finger. The official medical term is fibro-adenoma.

Over thirty the suspect lumps nearly always turn out to be cysts, also benign and containing fluid. So finding a lump nine times out of ten early on in the fertile years is going to prove harmless, but the great thing is to report immediately and have fears set at rest, *not* go on worrying and doing nothing.

Certainly the chances of a lump being more serious increases with age, and fifty-seven is the peak age for actual breast cancer. It cannot be emphasized too much that the earlier any such problem is found and tackled the better the chances of recovery. In this connection it does seem to me after talking to experts in this field, that women in this country should be pressing and pressing hard for much better provision of mammography services. This can reveal very very early onset of the disease, even before a lump can be felt by you or by the skilled fingers of a doctor doing a breast check by hand, officially called palpation.

Mammography is a painless X-ray technique reckoned to be 90 per cent accurate in diagnosing breast cancer. In fact, Professor A. P. Forest, now Regius Professor of Surgery at Edinburgh University Medical School, reported a 97 per cent diagnostic accuracy rate for benign and malignant breast lumps, using a combination of clinical examination and mammography, when working in the breast cancer clinic in Cardiff.[28]

Mr Geoffrey Oates, consultant surgeon to the United Birmingham Hospitals, told me:

I'm sure mammography should be much more widely used. Its effectiveness for diagnosis had been proven and in New York, where Dr Strax screened an enormous population, the pick-up of really early breast cancer by mammography was significantly better than simply from normal medical presentation.[29] By the time a lump is apparent, there will be systemic involvement with a chance of the cancer spreading elsewhere in around half the cases. With mammography it is possible to detect earlier before that happens.

As with so many life-saving medical advances, it's partly a matter of educating the public and partly a matter of sheer finance and priorities within the Health Service. In a sense public knowledge about these new techniques and their value can influence provision of finance and help determine priorities. At the moment the DHSS is only prepared to run some very modest pilot schemes on breast screening including mammography in just three or four centres, instead of setting up a national scheme which could save so much suffering and so many lives. Women and in particular influential Women's groups like the National Council of Women, WIs and Townswomen's Guilds have exerted considerable pressure for things like wider availability of HRT at the menopause, and this has had its effect. I believe they should now begin to exert real pressure for full breast-screening services to include mammography, now that the evidence for its value is accumulating.

It's encouraging in this connection that Marks & Spencer have now set up their own nationwide scheme of breast-screening with mammography, for all their women employees over the age of thirty-five.

Another method of diagnosis which has received quite a lot of publicity is thermography, which relies on picking up temperature changes in affected tissue. The newspapers particularly went to town on a rather experimental extension of this method involving a special bra, designed to register just such local temperature variations in the breast and so act as a continuous monitoring system. It has to be said that, although thermography and mapping the heat pattern of the breast does have some value – it is cheap and involves no X-ray exposure – it is really as yet far too inaccurate to be of proven worth in the way mammography is.

When a woman is referred to a specialist with a breast lump one of the first tests is usually with a needle. Needle aspiration of the breast, although accurate in most cases, still leaves some problems unresolved, and a recent leading article in the *BMJ* suggests that more work is needed before this can be depended on for the diagnosis of breast cancer. 'Getting the needle' does not usually have a pleasant connotation, but for between 60 and 70 per cent of women in their late thirties, it will bring immediate and overwhelming relief. They walk out of that clinic on air and with no scar on body or mind.

Protracted anxiety and uncertainty is hard to bear and another splendid new procedure is helping to reduce both. This is the use of a special biopsy needle where it is felt further investigation is warranted. With the needle a small core of tissue can be extracted and the specialist can get an exact diagnosis there and then, all done under a local anaesthetic, and enabling him to set the patient's fears at rest or to discuss further treatment with her if this is going to be necessary. This is a very new and valuable development, not yet used nearly widely enough, and involving what is called a Tru-cut needle.

The more conventional method of biopsy, used if clinical examination and mammography reveal a suspect hard lump or cluster of cells, is to remove the mass quickly under general anaesthetic, examine it microscopically by a procedure called a 'frozen section' and, if this reveals malignancy to proceed to fuller surgery.

In these cases the 'treatment of choice', as it has been rather ironically described, has tended to be radical surgery. This involves removal of the tumour and a good margin of surrounding tissue together with any affected glands, as cancer cells can migrate through the drainage system of the body as well as directly through the blood stream.

The trend now, however, is toward more conservative treatment, as there is absolutely no proof of greater value in what have been termed 'heroic' operations – the 'heroic' should perhaps have been applied to the patients!

Treatment of breast cancer is very much a team job. Good pathologists are essential for accurate diagnosing and grading of the malignancy, and good surgeons for the actual operation. But in addition to surgery there is also radiotherapy, hormone therapy and chemotherapy, and the real answer would seem to lie more and more with specialized centres and pools of expertise. There are already half a dozen or so such places in this country and many more are needed.

So much is being learned all the time. For example not long ago radiotherapy was almost automatic after mastectomy (removal of breast), but now the trend is more toward the 'wait-and-watch' system, since controlled trials have failed to show any great benefit to the groups treated with immediate radiation.

On the other hand chemotherapy as additional follow-up treatment is being increasingly used with some evidence of improved results. Reports from both America and Italy have shown quite a dramatic increase in survival rates,[30] and currently big trials are going on in this country, including some in the West Midlands, where various combinations of drugs are being tried on some groups after surgery and results compared with other groups having surgery alone.

Chemotherapy does have some unpleasant side-effects, including hair loss, which can be very distressing, though it is usually only a temporary side-effect, lasting during the treatment period. I asked Mr Oates if it was a great ethical trauma virtually playing at God and deciding which woman should have this drug treatment and which should not, in groups where the indications were equally valid. He replied:

We shall find no firm answers without controlled trials. This has slowed down progress in cancer treatment and assessment of results. In any case, we are not 'playing at God', as you put it, because we genuinely do not yet know whether chemotherapy is justified in these cases. We just know we have got to find out whether it does give a better survival rate over long periods. It appears to in the short term but that is not enough.

One other line of attack being studied in connection with breast cancer, as with other cancers, is concerned with the body's own immune mechanism. Work is going on all round the world and vast sums being poured into research. Men like

Dr Bernard Strehler, whom I met at the University of Southern California, are gradually unlocking the secrets of cell behaviour. Strehler believes both the ageing process and probably the mechanism underlying some forms of cancer involves the failing ability of cells to decode messages correctly. The eventual answer will almost certainly be found at the cellular level.

Meanwhile the most powerful weapon we have is early diagnosis and this is most especially true in dealing with cervical cancer.

Cervical cancer

Caught early enough cervical cancer is 100 per cent curable, so it is the more tragic that 1 per cent of British women still die of this disease, almost all of whom could have been saved by early and regular smear tests.

Joe Jordan is going to be embarrassed to find himself appearing rather frequently in these pages, but he is a leading consultant gynaecologist in Birmingham where I live and work and is always ready to help, advise and ensure my information is accurate. He is also the first-ever British doctor to be given the very prestigious appointment of president of the Pan American Cancer Cytology Society, and so his views on this subject have very special authority.

We know that the majority of deaths from cervical cancer are preventable, because this form of cancer goes through a pre-cancer stage that can be readily detected by smear tests. Once detected the abnormal cells can easily be removed or destroyed. All women who are sexually active should be having this test done regardless of age, and initially it should be repeated within one year. After that every two or three years is enough.

The reference to sexually active women being the ones at risk is based on a now acknowledged link between cervical cancer and sexual intercourse. This link was first suspected when it was found that the disease never occurred in virgins. In particular it was never found in nuns, except where there had been sexual experience before taking vows or a lapse afterwards.

In contrast to this negative evidence, positive evidence comes in the form of the very high incidence of cervical cancer found among prostitutes and also in women who started having inter-course at a very early age, or who were promiscuous.

The lining of the neck of the womb (cervix), particularly in the young, is thought to be susceptible to cancer-inducing agents, probably contained in the sperm itself or possibly in a sexually transmitted virus. A type of herpes virus, *not* the one that causes cold sores, but another known as H S V 2, has come under particular suspicion with high levels of antibodies to it being found both in women with cervical cancer and/or in their husbands.

Promiscuity in husbands can also be linked to the incidence of this disease in wives, as can a direct link between higher levels of venereal disease, particularly syphilis, in husbands and higher rates of cervical cancer in wives.

Strangely enough there is also a connection shown by two quite separate studies, both giving very similar figures, between the risk of cervical cancer in the wife and the husband's occupa-tion. The highest risk applies to the wives of manual workers, to wives of fishermen, seamen, labourers, lorry drivers, etc., who all have three or four times the chance of contracting cervical cancer compared to the wives of clerical workers, teachers, scientists, doctors, etc. The lowest rate of all applies to the wives of clergymen, and as it's unlikely they are blessed in this way simply because of their husband's calling, it re-inforces the distinct impression that neither the clergy nor their wives are promiscuous!

The earlier age of intercourse in many women, belonging to what used in the past to be termed the 'working class', may be involved in this. But with class differences diminishing and promiscuity increasing right across the board, it will be interest-ing to see if future studies show a similar disparity of risk.

Meanwhile it cannot be emphasized too strongly that *none* of these factors need to be involved at all. The risk factor is present anyway for *all* women who have intercourse, so that ordinary married women leading normal and virtuous married lives still incur some degree of unavoidable risk, and the discovery of the pre-cancerous and treatable condition or of cervical cancer itself carries absolutely no stigma and is no reflection on life-style. It is just that the more sexual partners a woman may have the more chance she also has of one of them being what is known as a 'high risk male'. But equally the one partner she does have may fall into this category and in his case too there may be no connection whatever with his sex life but only with a special type of sperm.

This concept of some men having a higher risk than others of somehow inducing cervical cancer, and a link with a special type of sperm, is the basis of some of the most interesting work being done in this field. In this country the man heavily involved in this research is Dr Albert Singer, senior lecturer in the Department of Obstetrics and Gynaecology at the University of Sheffield.[31] Dr Singer told me:

A recent study based on work in Baltimore showed that men whose first wives had cervical cancer seem to carry the higher risk with them when they marry again, and the second wives too show a higher incidence. Bevan Reid in Australia and myself have been interested in the possibility that a certain type of sperm is involved. In particular we have been looking at the coating around these sperm. This seems to be made up of basic proteins called 'histones' and it seems the same coating surrounds the H S V 2 virus. Histones have a profound effect on the surface of the cervix cell, disrupting its cellular mechanism. Animal work by other teams has already confirmed this and shown the tumour-inducing potential of histones.

Dr Singer went on the explain that he and Dr Reid were checking histone variations, in particular the higher levels in the sperm and semen of some men which would, on this theory, obviously increase the risk of inducing cancer.

One starting point is the man known to have been having sexual intercourse with a young woman who develops the disease. At sixteen, for instance, a girl cannot yet have had many sexual partners, and we find some presenting perhaps with venereal disease and within a short time the pre-cancerous condition of the cervix also shows up. So it is not difficult then to trace and examine sperm of the man involved.

Dr Singer and Bevan Reid have already won the René Moricard Prize for work on cervical cancer, and the implications of histone may well go beyond cervical cancer into other genital and female cancers. If and when the high risk male can be identified, obviously special steps would be taken to use protective barrier methods of contraception, and to keep wives and sexual partners very carefully screened.

As already pointed out the *pre*-cancerous state is readily detectable by a cervical smear. It is also readily treatable and, in the past, the first step has always been what is called a cone biopsy, very minor surgery, but still requiring a general anaesthetic and a short stay in hospital. Afterwards further checks must be done regularly to make sure no abnormal cells remain or recur. If by any chance they do, the only course to ensure safety was once a hysterectomy, regardless of age.

Now, however, it is exciting to report yet another tremendous advance. Both to treat the initial pre-cancerous condition and to treat any residual cancer following conventional cone biopsy, a special laser has been developed. Lasers have been associated in the public mind more with death than life – with killing rather than healing – representing the nearest science-fact has managed to get to the science-fiction concept of a death ray. But this new special life-giving laser is being increasingly used to destroy the diseased cells and save women from muti-lating surgery.

The first to be brought to this country and already in action here is at the Birmingham Women's Hospital. Joe Jordan told me how he came to introduce the system here. 'Lasers are already available in a few medical centres in the States,' he explained, 'being used most successfully to treat women suffer-ing from pre-cancer of the cervix or recurrent cancer of the cervix. I was able to see how the system worked while I was over there lecturing at the University of Wisconsin Medical School. I became determined that British women too should have the benefit, so I took the chance to study it and arranged for a machine to be sent over.'

It was a courageous decision because the laser itself cost £17000 and at that time Mr Jordan had no idea how it could be paid for in the present state of the NHS. 'I felt the important thing was to get the laser over, into use and demonstrate its enormous benefit,' he insisted. 'Then I reckoned I'd face the problem of how to fund it. I've great faith in the generosity of people for something like this.'

His faith proved justified, when a Birmingham business man, John Coleman, read about the laser and its work, sent a cheque for the full £17000, and another reader, a Mrs Willetts, sent a further £5000 for the rather special colposcope used in conjunction with the laser. This is an instrument which enables the doctor to look right at the cervix down a special eye-piece and pinpoint the diseased cells. The colposcope used with the laser also permits the laser beam to travel down a parallel path to focus on the cells and literally burn them out and destroy them.

One of Mr Jordan's patients, Jennifer Baker, was full of praise for the laser treatment. Earlier conventional treatment at her local hospital had still left residual pre-cancerous cells, and at thirty-five with only one child the prospect of a hysterectomy was not very welcome. She told me, 'You don't feel any pain at all with the laser treatment, but best of all you don't have to stay in hospital, and being an out-patient takes all the fear and dread out of it.'

Thanks to the laser a hysterectomy has been avoided for Jennifer, and she will be able to go on to have other children if she wants to do so. The great hope of this new laser technique, once it gets known, is that it will encourage more women to come forward for the simple test, and if necessary what now can be only simple out-patient treatment, not only to save life, but in the long run to save the NHS money.

Even in the short time the laser has been in use at Birmingham its effectiveness has been proven and its economy too. Mr Jordan emphasized this in his hopes for future expansion. 'I'd like to see each major centre in the UK with its own laser and a team trained to use it,' he told me. 'We're already setting up training courses. By avoiding more radical and more expensive in-patient care, we estimate that in just the first five out-patient sessions we saved the NHS £7000.'

Savings on that scale will soon pay for a crop of lasers and hopefully Mr Jordan's hopes will be realized for wider availability across the country.* But meanwhile it is still vital for women to come forward for that simple, quick and painless initial smear test. Of every 1000 smears done, about twenty show some abnormal cells, but on further check only three of

* Already a second laser has been ordered and, by the time this book comes out, will be operative at the Queen Mother's Hospital, Glasgow. What is more, it has been paid for this time by the NHS!

these actually prove to require further examination and perhaps treatment. The great thing to remember is that at this
stage it is 100 per cent curable.

Cancer of the uterus

Cancer of the uterus or body of the womb is less common than
cancer of the cervix and usually found in older women, the high
risk age being between fifty and sixty. Unfortunately the simple
smear test does not readily detect this, and so doctors must rely
on women having the sense to report symptoms. Any woman
who develops irregular bleeding after the age of thirty-five
should see her doctor. It will almost invariably prove to be due
to hormonal changes, but just occasionally it may be the first
and early sign of cancer of the womb. It is even more important
to report and deal with this promptly if it occurs after the
menopause. However scanty the bleeding the doctor should be
told. The only exception is what is termed the 'scheduled'
bleeding, predictable and expected during the week off therapy
in women on HRT, particularly under the new safest system
which uses the combined therapy including a progestogen, and
is positively designed to produce a regular monthly bleed.

Bleeding at any other time must be reported even in women
on HRT. Luckily cancer of the womb grows only very slowly,
so that if a woman follows this advice it is generally curable by
hysterectomy (removal of the womb) and this is discussed in
detail later in this chapter.

Cancer of the ovaries

About 5 per cent of cancers in women occur in the ovary, so
that it is not one of the most common forms, which is just as
well as it is not easy to detect. All women over forty should have
a periodic pelvic examination, as the only clue to possible
ovarian cancer is enlargement of the ovary which the doctor
can feel. Even then 95 per cent of such ovarian abnormality is
non-cancerous, but usually in the older women to be on the safe
side removal of the affected ovary (called an oopherectomy) or
even both ovaries is recommended. Again this is discussed in
conjunction with hysterectomy a little later in this chapter.

Cancer of the vulva

Happily this is very rare and found principally in much older women. Any elderly women who have persistent vulval itch should seek medical attention, and to exclude early cancer a tiny piece of skin is removed under a local anaesthetic quite painlessly.

Younger women may often notice small growths on the vulva and fortunately these are almost always benign, but they should just be checked. Itchiness during the fertile years is also almost always due to other non-serious causes and these are discussed later.

Meanwhile, as with cervical cancer, cancer of the vulva is usually preceded by a pre-malignancy stage. Detected early, the treatment is relatively simple with a very good chance of success. But ignored and allowed to progress to what is termed invasive cancer, then the surgery is much more extensive and the outlook far less good.

Hysterectomy and oopherectomy

Hysterectomy is the removal of the womb and it comes in a variety of forms, but by the age of seventy-five some 19 per cent of women will have had one form or other of this surgery.

For any woman the removal of her womb and possibly one or both of her ovaries (oopherectomy) is a traumatic experience emotionally as well as physically. She's losing the part of her body that has carried and nourished her children, the part that she may feel makes her specially female. While doctors argue that for the woman who has completed her family the womb is no longer of any use and may as well be removed, many women fear it will all lead to premature menopause, accelerated ageing, adverse effects on sex life and a high risk of depression.

At one time a great many of these fears were justified. But today with HRT available and almost routinely used, certainly where ovaries have been removed, none of these dreaded things will happen.

Recent surveys have certainly confirmed that in untreated women, not given HRT, depression is four times as common in women who have had ovaries removed as in other women. It is also more severe and of longer duration, and one of the studies by Dr D. H. Richards, carried out in Oxford, also showed increased depression following even simple hysterectomy. This is believed to be due to the ovaries working less efficiently in cases where surgery may have interfered with the normal blood supply.

This new understanding of the effect of even simple hysterectomy means really that there should be good and sufficient reason for the operation, and that it should not be used, as it has sometimes been in the past, as the easy way out – easy for the doctors, not so easy for the woman. There is a feeling, applying more strongly perhaps to the American medical scene than the British, that knife-happy surgeons have been too ready to remove symptoms by removing the uterus, without properly establishing the cause and considering the alternative of controlling heavy bleeding, for instance, by use of hormones.

Now, of course, where excessive bleeding or discharge is due to uterine disease, or where there are large fibroids, there is no alternative to surgery, and at least use of HRT means today that no woman needs to dread awful after-effects.

One decision for the surgeon to make is whether the hysterectomy, when necessary, should be sub-total which involves only removal of the womb, or total which includes removal of the head of the cervix. Also of course he has to decide whether the ovaries can be safely left.

Where a hysterectomy is really necessary, there is a strongish case for *total* hysterectomy, as this precludes any possibility of cervical cancer developing at a later stage.

The decision about the ovaries is far more difficult, and the age of the patient and the reason for the hysterectomy as well as the state of the ovaries themselves are vital determining factors.

If the ovaries are diseased, of course, then however young the woman may be they need to be removed. If the ovaries appear healthy but there is a past history of ovarian cancer in the family, then again most gynaecologists would consider they should be removed. Any increasing pre-menopausal hirsuitism (hairiness) suggesting abnormal ovarian function would also be an indication for removal, to be followed up with high dosages of oestrogen.

Finally, many surgeons would also remove ovaries when carrying out a hysterectomy on any woman over forty-five, on the assumption that the ovary's useful life is almost over at that age, and so, as with the cervix, they are removing just another possible seat of future cancer.

Against this, other doctors argue that normal-looking ovaries should be conserved where possible, even in women of this age or just over. They insist that the ovaries continue to work in some women for several years beyond the initial onset of the menopause and even beyond final menstruation. One way of checking this would be a vaginal smear just before the operation, which would help to confirm the oestrogen level and if this indicated only poor ovarian function, then there would obviously be less reason to leave them.

The method by which hysterectomies are done also affects the question of removal of ovaries. They are far more likely to be conserved when a vaginal hysterectomy is done (removing the womb through the vagina as the name implies). With an abdominal one, not only can the ovaries be seen and inspected but of course removed very simply.

So the decision finally has to be based on medical judgement, but at least women should know what is involved and the various alternatives, so that they can understand the situation and be sure that both judgement and knowledge are used properly on their behalf, and that surgery is not simply seen as the easy way out.

Many women following a hysterectomy, particularly with treatment if oestrogen deficiency symptoms show up, can take on a new lease of life and there can be a very positive and constructive side to what women still tend to call '*the* operation'. With modern hormone treatment available when needed, there does not need to be any 'castrating' effect even when ovaries are removed; it does not shorten the vagina to make sexual intercourse difficult; it does not make a woman less desirable or less responsive and nor does it lead to obesity. The younger the woman subjected to this surgery, the more important it is for her to be sure to get HRT treatment.

There is strong evidence that when the ovaries are removed early in life, women become four times more at risk from heart disease. To prevent this, and to prevent severe menopause problems and increased risk of osteoparosis, very often today an oestrogen implant is given at the time of surgery and renewed as needed or replaced by oral oestrogen. With the uterus removed there is no problem of bleeding on HRT and no need for a progestogen to be added. Another very obvious bonus, of course, is that contraception is no longer necessary, so there are several pluses and, with modern surgical techniques, modern pain relief and HRT, old fears can be forgotten.

Menstrual disorders

Chapter 3 dealt with one aspect of this subject, and we have also briefly touched on the effect of the emotions on menstruation, particularly in causing temporary failure of periods.

But there can be other causes to disturb hormone levels and trigger irregular or heavy menstrual bleeding, and these days appropriate hormone treatment can usually correct the problem. To exclude other reasons, such as polyps, however, a diagnostic curettage is usually done; this is colloquially known as a 'scrape' and medically as a D and C.

D and C

This stands for 'dilation and curettage' and is a very simple procedure in which the cervix is gently dilated to allow the gynaecologist to scrape the lining of the womb. From this cells are examined. A general anaesthetic is used, but only a very brief stay of one night in hospital needed.

Vabra curettage

This is another method increasingly used just to obtain a sample of the lining of the womb, so that again cells can be checked for any abnormality. It is done as an out-patient procedure, takes only a few minutes and is only slightly uncomfortable involving not even a local anaesthetic. With the recognition of the importance of regular screening, this is an economic and useful development, again saving time, money and in-patient care.

Fibroids

This is a very common female problem and is non-malignant, rarely proceeding to become so. About twenty-five out of every 100 women develop fibroids by the time they are forty years of age, and they often cause an increased menstrual flow and increased duration of loss, due to their enlargement of the uterine cavity. If a fibroid encroaches on the lining of the womb, it tends to cause spotty bleeding and may prevent pregnancy or cause recurrent spontaneous abortion.

Most fibroids cause neither pain nor symptoms but because of their tendency to grow, there should be regular follow-up and this applies particularly to the older woman on HRT (oestrogen may stimulate fibroids) and equally for the same reason to the younger woman on the contraceptive pill.

Polyps

These again are rarely malignant and are really just little glandular bags of tissue which can also cause irregular bleeding. If they are in the cervix they can be removed easily and painlessly as an out-patient procedure. If within the womb itself, then a D and C may be required.

Vaginal discharge

A degree of vaginal discharge is normal and usually healthy. The natural secretions not only keep the vagina moist but clean. Some women on some contraceptive pills get increased discharge and so do many women at the time of ovulation. Although it is a very common reason for women consulting their doctors, unless the discharge is irritating there is almost certainly no real problem.

But certain vaginal infections can cause irritation and these should be treated.

Vaginal infections

Trichomonas

This is the most common with 10 per cent of women carrying this organism. It can remain dormant for years producing no symptoms, or it can flare up to cause inflammation and itching of the vulva, vagina and a greenish discharge. Fortunately these days excellent treatments are available on prescription, and a course of tablets, often together with creams or pessaries, will rapidly relieve the discomfort and the infection. Because the husband too may be a carrier, though almost always without any symptoms at all, it is really wise for him too to receive a course of tablets and so prevent re-infection during intercourse.

Monilia (Thrush)

This again is a very common form of infection caused by a yeast organism rather like a fungus. It also produces itching and burning, but the secretion with monilia is more like a white curd. Again it can be present without causing symptoms. Sometimes, while on an antibiotic for other reasons, monilia will flare up as the antibiotic also kills off the protective bacteria which normally keep it at bay.

Women troubled by recurrent monilia should avoid nylon knickers which tend to retain moisture. Again good treatments now exist in similar form to those used for Trichomas with special anti-yeast creams, pessaries and tablets. Again if the problem keeps recurring, the husband may also be a carrier and a check should be done to establish this and if necessary he should be treated too.

Vaginal infections of this kind can be very miserable and really affect the quality of life, so the important thing is to remember that good treatment is now possible. A splendid preparation called nystatin became available during the last decade, and more recently another very effective one called Daktarin (miconazole nitrate) is proving of enormous help in dealing with this minor but literally irritating condition.

Urinary tract infections

Cystitis or bladder infection causes enormous misery to vast numbers of women. It is more common in women, as are all sorts of urinary infections, because the urethra (the stem of the bladder) is much shorter in women and does not offer such a good barrier against infection as the longer one of the male.

The opening of the urethra is also close to the vagina and may be bruised during sexual intercourse (this leads to what is sometimes called 'honeymoon cystitis'). It is also near the anus (back-passage) which makes it rather open to germs from the intestinal tract.

The aftermath of having babies such as scarring or cystocele (prolapse of the bladder) can also add to the risk of infections of this kind. Some doctors also insist that women simply do not drink enough water either, and this allows the urine in the bladder to stagnate and the bacteria to proliferate.

The symptoms are the need to pass urine frequently and pain in the process. The water may be cloudy and sometimes there can even be traces of blood present. Simply taking a specimen in any old bottle is really not sufficient, as these days to identify the actual infection for more specific treatment doctors like a mid-stream specimen in a sterile container and this is best done at the surgery or clinic.

The majority of urinary infections in women come from the bowel and the urine is tested and cultured to find out just what bacteria is involved. Fortunately these days antibiotics and sulfa drugs are available and effective. For one special type of infection caused by the *E. coli* bacteria a new drug called Selexid is particularly good. The *E. coli* normally lives happily in the bowel, causing no trouble and doing its job of dealing with waste matter.

But if for any reason it manages to get into the urinary tract it can give rise to miserable symptoms and inflammation. Drugs such as Septrin led the way to a series of new drugs which have the advantage of being selective in their action, really decimating the straying *E. coli*, and they are particularly useful in resistant cases.

Chronic or repeatedly recurring cystitis should always be fully investigated and a cystoscopy with a simple examination of the inside of the bladder may be advisable. It is very important for this condition to be treated and a final urine analysis carried out to make sure any infection has been cleared.

Perhaps more emphasis should be placed on prevention, and this can involve both drinking more fluid and correct hygiene, with cleansing from front to back to avoid the risk of bowel germs getting wiped in the wrong direction.

Pubic lice

This really sounds a very off-putting subject but unhappily the fact remains that these tiny crab-like creatures can be caught by any one of us simply from infested towels, bedding or clothing. They can also, of course, be sexually transmitted and so are on the increase along with all other sexually transmittable diseases in this more sexually active society we live in.

The pubic or 'crab' lice clasp the hair with their hind claws, making them difficult to dislodge and they bite into the skin in order to feed on blood. The females lay about eight eggs a day and cement them to the foot of the hairs with the nits hatching out in about one week. The lice can sometimes penetrate to the hair under the armpits or even eyebrows and eyelashes, but *never* to the scalp.

Fortunately today there is extremely effective treatment. Shaving the pubic hair is not necessary and lotions, ointments and shampoos containing a substance called gamma benzene hexachloride work rapidly. Prioderm is one effective form, sold both as lotion and shampoo, and if instructions are followed the condition can be cleared with one treatment, though a follow-up is advised in a week to ten days as a further form of insurance. The infestation produces a slight itching which may be the only symptom to alert anyone and they should not only deal at once with their own problem but of course change bedding and warn anyone else with whom they may have been in intimate contact. Obviously unless both sexual partners clear the infestation, they can re-infect each other.

Gonorrhoea

This is the most common form of venereal disease and in fact is reported as being more common than measles today in the Western world. This can only be sexually transmitted and it is even more important to see that any sexual contacts are warned to help prevent the spread.

The problem with gonorrhoea is that in the early stages the symptoms may be so slight that they can be overlooked. Usually in a woman there is a slight burning during urination for a few days usually followed by subsidence of this symptom. This can mean a spontaneous cure but it can also mean the bacteria causing the disease have just lodged in the mouth of the uterus where they may remain dormant for years but produce serious problems later. Gonorrhoea can affect the Bartholin gland to produce abscesses; it may produce inflammation of the vagina or even in some cases spread up through the womb into the fallopian tubes to produce a severe illness with high fever, abdominal pain and vaginal discharge of pus. This is called gonorrhoeal salpingitis and is usually first noticed a few days after a menstrual period, because the menstrual blood helps the bacteria to breed.

Although fortunately gonorrhoea responds to modern antibiotics, it is estimated some 13 per cent of women lose their fertility even after just one severe attack if it involves the fallopian tubes.

Men can carry the bacteria in their prostate glands after an acute attack and be unaware of its presence, just as woman may be unaware if it is dormant in the cervix.

Because of the rising incidence anyone who might have been exposed or women having multiple sexual partners should have regular cervical and urethral cultures performed. We have splendid VD clinics now in this country and there is a clear responsibility for anyone with symptoms or suspecting contact to get the infection dealt with. Usually the bacteria can be killed off by a single treatment, but not all gonorrhoea germs are exactly the same. Some strains initially resist treatment and because of this everyone should make certain to have follow-up tests to check the cure is complete. The serious complications can be avoided by early diagnosis and treatment, so any unusual vaginal discharge should always be investigated or a burning sensation when passing water or symptoms of fever, chill, abdominal pain and painful joints.

A male sexual partner can usually detect if he has the problem again by pain on passing water, or yellow discharge from the penis. Men can help prevent the disease in themselves by using a sheath; urinating and washing after intercourse also helps. For women prevention is more difficult. Again the old-fashioned barrier contraception offers some protection, but otherwise her best protection must be in knowledge of her partner and trust in his sense of responsibility to her. Inspection of the penis can reveal ulcers or skin rash which can also be symptoms in the male, but of syphilis rather than gonorrhoea.

Syphilis

Like gonorrhoea this more serious form of venereal disease is also becoming more prevalent as a result of increased sexual activity in the younger generation and the use of modern oral contraceptives or IUDs rather than sheaths.

The only sign of early infection in a woman is a small ulcer, usually on the cervix or in the vagina. These ulcers have what is termed a 'punched-out' appearance and are usually painless, though they sometimes give off a bloody discharge. Again, of course, a microbe is responsible and again it enters the body through sexual intercourse. If the original sores heal over the disease can still be detected because after two or three weeks the germs will have entered the blood stream and will show up in a blood test. After an incubation period a red spot appears on the skin where the germ entered and a hard, painless but typical syphilis chancre appears. Ninety-five per cent of them are on or near the genital areas but patients can be unaware of them, particularly if they are inside the vagina. After a few weeks or months, however, a widespread rash occurs. Some people develop enough antibodies for a cure to take place naturally, but for the other 50 per cent the disease can progress if untreated to a final serious stage involving disfigurement and even death.

Again it is absolutely essential to seek early diagnosis and treatment if there is the slightest suspicion of having the disease or having been in contact with it. Syphilis germs are extremely sensitive to penicillin, to tetracycline and other antibiotics, but a longer course is needed than for gonorrhoea. Again the follow-up is vital to ensure a proper cure has been achieved. And remember that while early syphilis *can* be cured, it becomes really serious if untreated and spreads disaster not only to sexual partners but in women to their unborn babies, who may be born dead or suffer later from deafness or blindness. With our good network of VD clinics in this country and good treatment available, this disease should never be allowed to get on the increase.

11. New relationships

Having looked now at the female facts of life, pleasant and unpleasant, together with the new medical lifelines being offered to us, it seems to me that in this last chapter we should consider how the new freedoms these confer, and our growing confidence in ourselves as women, may affect our relationships and attitudes to others, ourselves and doctors.

Their most important influence of course, must be on our sexual lives. Many complete books have already been written on this complex subject and obviously I cannot deal with it fully in just one chapter. For those wanting more detailed information, I have listed some recent books in the bibliography at the back.

The availability of effective contraception in the last few decades, superimposed on the weakening of religious and social sanctions, have virtually swept away the wretched double standards which once, so illogically, expected all nice girls to remain virgins until marriage while decreeing that the nice men they would ultimately marry should somehow be sexually experienced. The only obvious answer was two types of women – those who wouldn't for love or money, and those who would for either or neither.

That has largely changed and, with contraception enabling women to separate the act of love from procreation, as men have always managed to do, women have begun to appreciate their own sexual natures and their capacity to receive pleasure as well as to give it.

But new freedoms bring new pressures and problems. At one time a woman could refuse a full sexual relationship with the strong and valid excuse of a fear of pregnancy and of social stigma. Today (except in rare cases where religious scruples still apply) the only reason she can give for refusing is that she simply does not want the man to make love to her, and it is a reason male vanity finds hard to accept or forgive.

The reasons that lie *behind* the reason may be more complex in reality, varying from the simple failure of that particular hunk of male chemistry to turn her on, to her own fears of inadequacy or failure, or even to the belief, still deeply rooted in the female, that sex (and the giving and taking involved) is part of something called love and commitment, rather than lust and opportunism.

I believe that, despite all the liberation and the new morality, many woman retain a basically different attitude toward sex, built in by long conditioning. Over the centuries, indeed really until the last twenty or thirty years, sexual intercourse for a woman *had* to be a more serious matter than for a man. She might enjoy it. She might yield and be carried away against all her better judgement, but unless she was an idiot or totally irresponsible, she usually knew that there might be a day of reckoning, approximately nine months away.

Because of this possible consequence, the chances were that if she did make love, it was because her emotions were involved. This could well have led to the familiar chicken and egg situation (appropriate terminology in this particular context), so that a degree of emotional content and involvement became actually bred into female sexuality and response, in a way which did not apply to the male. So, for a lot of women sexual response remains far more complex than just an automatic, hormonal or largely mechanical business, set up by friction between penis and clitoris. Up to now for most women it has also included emotional overtones.

It has to be seen whether the wider availability of contraception, separating sex from procreation, will ultimately enable women to adopt the male attitude and the simpler male response. And it also remains to be seen whether it will, in the long run, prove a good thing for the human race.

Already there is some evidence that over-high expectations on the part of women, even a degree of female sexual aggression, may be having an emasculating effect on men, whose own anxiety about their ability to please and satisfy sometimes results in actual impotence. It would be an irony if rising female appreciation of sex inadvertently led to diminished opportunity.

Sexual harmony seems easier to attain if the woman's drive is equal to or greater than the man's; otherwise a man tends to compensate by looking elsewhere. A woman, through the emotional outlet offered by her children and home, can often sublimate sexual frustration less dangerously. Doctors do admit, however, that some women are giving expression to the problem of sexual incompatibility through various gynaecological symptoms such as excessive vaginal discharge, menstrual disorders or even plain backache and headache.

On the other hand, an unexpected and delightful by-product of the greater freedom today is the very real friendship that now seems to develop between young men and women *before* marriage, and a demand for that same friendship and companionship *within* marriage. Young men want and expect to marry a woman who will be very much more than a sexual object or a housekeeper. They expect her to be fun to live with. Young women need neither protector nor provider, but they do need a lover and a good mate in the wider and companionable sense of that word.

Down the centuries aphrodisiacs have been tried as a means of improving libido – oysters, for example. In our western society, of course, alcohol is the great erotic stimulant, but the best aphrodisiac for any woman is to be desired. The good lover, of course, knows this and takes the time and trouble to make the woman aware and aroused before attempting coitus. The neat word for sexual intercourse comes from the Latin, *coitio*, meaning literally 'go together'. But to 'go together' really well may take some time. Full sexual compatibility in many cases is only achieved with privacy, security and time to get to know each other's likes and dislikes. For these reasons, for the woman at any rate, the average casual sexual encounter, hurried, under tension, and perhaps without tenderness, can spell disaster and leave her disillusioned either with sex or perhaps, mistakenly, with her own capacity for sex, duped into believing she is unnatural and frigid. The first experience is particularly important, because first penetration can sometimes be painful. It helps for a woman to be aware of this and prepared for some bleeding, but it helps even more if the man is considerate, patient and gentle, all of which demands at least a caring relationship.

By no means all women do experience orgasm, despite all the lurid prose recently written about this aspect of sex. Even those who do normally reach a climax find that sometimes it eludes them or the man is too quick. It is obviously splendidly rewarding and releasing if it does happen and, once satisfactorily achieved, the sheer anticipation of pleasure plays its own part in the arousal mechanism, encouraging repetition. But it is important not to treat it as a major disaster if orgasm does not always happen, even more not to make a great thing about it happening at the same time as the male orgasm. Achieving a climax simultaneously can be a marvellous experience, but so can giving sexual pleasure to each other at different times and in different ways. Coitus is not the only acceptable and enjoyable sexual experience.

The researches of Dr William Masters and Virginia Johnson have done a great deal to demolish a lot of old nonsense in this respect. In particular they proved that the size of the penis has little bearing on whether a man can satisfy his partner, and that there is no physiological difference between orgasm achieved by coitus and one achieved by other stimulation. They also proved that many post-menopausal women continue to have good sexual drive. In cases where there were problems, they found hormone replacement of great value.

Whether at the menopause or earlier in life, any woman who finds sexual intercourse painful should seek medical advice. There may be a logical and simple reason for the pain, which hormones or other treatment can overcome. But if not, then there may be emotional problems leading to a subconscious tensing through fear of pregnancy, guilt or just plain distaste for the whole business, usually *inculcated* in some way during childhood. In such cases counselling or just talking about it can often help.

It would be a mistake to suggest that love-making is so complicated and fraught with problems that everyone needs to make a prolonged study of it, or that textbooks are necessary to perfect techniques. But it is equally naïve to believe, as my own generation often did, that it was just a question of 'doing what comes naturally' and everything would be all right. For some people it is, and the well-matched pair who have no problems from the start are fortunate. But for others it may require patience, tolerance, tenderness and even some deliberate attempts to vary techniques and find ways and means that mutually delight.

Frank discussion of sex between partners, both its pleasures and its problems, can be tremendously helpful and often stimulating, and it should be possible ideally without any feeling of embarrassment or shame. I have to confess it was very difficult indeed for women of my pre-war generation with our somewhat restrictive upbringing, and one of the bonuses of the present more open approach to sex is that young people today do seem able to to talk about it to each other far more easily and naturally. This must both enhance the pleasures and ease the problems.

Sometimes, even today, lack of sexual harmony can be rooted in an upbringing which has instilled the idea, usually in a daughter, that sex is evil or in some way dirty. Even refusing to answer a child's natural questions or punishing him or her for masturbation or touching the genital area, can warp sexuality and reduce sex drive in adult life. Masturbation for both sexes is perfectly normal, part of growing up, and three-quarters of women have used this method of sexual satisfaction by the age of twenty-one.

Many widely different cultures have seen masturbation as a means of learning or acquiring sexual function. Today in our own society, perhaps for the first time ever, there is some acceptance of this particularly among doctors specializing in sexual problems. There is some evidence that the woman who learns to masturbate and reach orgasm in this way will be better able to do so later in normal intercourse – one doctor likened the process to 'tuning up an engine' – hardly romantic but at least practical! In fact as opportunities of heterosexual contacts increase, masturbation usually decreases, but even if it does not there should be no feeling of guilt. It is not harmful – it does not damage eyesight, lead to acne, brain decay, insanity or venereal disease. These are old myths too long perpetuated by ignorance.

Neither with masturbation nor with conventional intercourse is it possible to lay down norms for frequency or intensity. Just as people have different appetites for food or drink and different capacities, so they have different levels of sex drive and need.

What is far more important is that the *relative* sex drive between two people hoping to sustain a long-term relationship should match reasonably well.

Just as women are beginning to realize that an intelligent approach to their relationships with men may well prove more rewarding and long-lasting than escapist romanticism, so they are also beginning to realize that they may well benefit from a better understanding of their own bodies and the way they function. This book will, I hope, have helped women in this and shown them how they can learn to be in control, instead of being dominated by, the mysteries of their own bodies.

In the past, doctors tended to encourage a lack of knowledge and an air of mystery as an aid to their profession. For the truth is, until the last few decades, medicine was far more of an art than a science, with largely ineffective drugs, and quite often harmful techniques. It had little but magic and mystique to offer. The more ignorant the patient, the more blind his faith in the wise healer, the more impressed he was by the coloured lotions, potions and mumbo-jumbo, the better the chance of aiding nature and speeding recovery through confidence and charisma.

Today things are entirely different. If the art of medicine required an ignorant and inert patient, the science of medicine in contrast requires an informed and cooperative patient. The increasing complexity of medicine demands real partnership between doctor and patient.

It has to be said that we are not always achieving this. Far from meriting the term 'partnership', it's doubtful if even the description 'relationship' can be justified, when in some busy group practices or clinics, all a patient may see of the doctor is a pair of eyes peering briefly over the ever-ready prescription pad, and when those eyes may not even belong to the same doctor twice running.

If that sounds a harsh comment, perhaps I should quickly add that it only describes one end of the spectrum and applies only to some areas and some practices. At the other extreme there are still dedicated doctors who somehow manage never to seem in a hurry, and between them are the great majority of GPs, striving to do the best they can within the confines of a system which often allows them only five minutes'

appointment time per patient in the normal surgery context.
But if there is lack of communication not all the fault lies
with the doctor. The patient, consciously or even subconsciously
responding to the pressure of the crowded waiting room and
perhaps already flustered and nervous, can all too easily fail to
mention the very symptoms which would most help their doctor
and outside the door again realize the *real* problem has never
been discussed.

Not all doctors agree with me but I believe this situation
applies rather more to women than to men. Women on the
whole seem to me to be too much in awe of their doctors, too
inarticulate in describing their problems, too apologetic for the
trouble they are causing. So many of the letters they write to
me are full of a sort of apologetic despair, as though the whole
thing were somehow their fault instead of their misfortune. Just
occasionally the attitude of their doctor has reinforced this
feeling. One woman wrote:

> I'm an ordinary NHS patient and far from being hypochondriac.
> I've rarely visited my doctor over the years except when I was
> having my three babies. Yet now with the menopause making me
> feel tired and depressed, with flushes and sweats making life a
> misery, he tells me that it's all in the mind and only the neurotic
> woman cannot cope with something that is natural. My husband
> puts great faith in medical advice, and if the doctor says there's
> nothing wrong with me, my husband believes him. It has made
> me feel guilty but I still can't believe it's natural to feel so ill.

A great many women report doctors reaching for their prescription pad almost before they've had time to describe symptoms or mention the headaches, depression or irritability. A
rapid prescription for librium, valium or pain-killers to treat
the symptoms is easier and quicker than the longer talk or
deeper investigation needed to establish the underlying cause.
One middle-aged woman from Essex wrote:

> I tried to tell my doctor I'd felt upside down ever since my
> periods had stopped eight years ago. I wanted to tell him about the
> hairs around my mouth and chin, about intercourse being so painful
> and my marriage becoming a mess, but he more or less cut me short
> by saying it was only the change and he had really sick people to
> attend to. I felt more depressed than ever and was sent away with a
> prescription for valium which makes me like a zombie.

Recent studies have shown that vast quantities of tranquil-lizers and anti-depressants are being prescribed for middle-aged woman, and it was irritating to see these statistics recently cited by a well-known doctor as proof that women are more neurotic than men. In fact they are only proof that doctors believe women to be more neurotic, and that this is the only medication they are usually offered for conditions which may often have a hormonal basis and a hormonal cure. The mistaken belief that medical care under the NHS is somehow a *free* service, almost a form of charity, can underly the tentative or over-apologetic approach. We need to remind ourselves (if our diminished pay packet does not already do so) that the NHS is far from free. We pay heavily for all our medical, social and welfare services, both in direct and indirect taxation and through National Insurance deductions.

Nothing, of course, can ever pay for that extra special care over and above the call of duty which many dedicated doctors still manage to give, but in the more routine sense we owe our doctors only normal respect, courtesy and cooperation. That means taking note of his views but not treating them as infallible; it means after agreeing a course of treatment doing our best to carry it out; after making an appointment doing our best to keep it punctually; and finally being as considerate as possible in asking for house-calls, and avoiding night time and weekend except in real emergency.

And the *quid pro quo*, of course, is that our doctors should also respect us and return the courtesy, using a realistic appoint-ments system, which does not involve insupportable delays when we may already be feeling less than well, or presumably we wouldn't be in the doctor's waiting room. It also means taking the time to listen to us and sometimes asking just the right question to elicit the underlying problem which some patients, particularly patients of the opposite sex, can be too shy to articulate without a little encouragement. And it also means where decisions have to be made, explaining the balance of risk and benefit and involving the patient in the ultimate choice of action.

We have to get rid of fear on the part of some patients and feudalism on the part of some doctors. Most of my examples seem to come from women striving to get HRT or treatment for PMS, but they still reveal these old attitudes and the implicit obedience some doctors expect from patients. One woman told me, 'My doctor not only refused to consider giving me oestrogen despite terrible flushes day and night, but actually said, "I forbid you to go elsewhere," when I asked to be referred. He was in a towering rage about it all and I dare not tell him now that I have been privately. It will be hopeless if the gynaecologist insists on contacting him.'

So in the doctor's authoritarianism and in the woman's timidity lay the root of bad doctoring, because the GP should *always* be informed of any special treatment a patient is receiving from a consultant and exactly what drugs she is on.

Other letters reported women being made to feel guilty for daring to read newspaper reports and idiots for believing them. Articles tentatively shown to doctors were flung into waste paper baskets and on one occasion my *No Change* was hurled across the surgery and the poor woman told she could choose between Wendy Cooper or her doctor. One woman wrote to me in great distress:

My doctor was so furious when he found out I had gone privately for HRT that he told me I must find another doctor. He would no longer keep me on his list. I don't mind for myself because I feel I have lost faith in him since the treatment he refused to give me has got rid so rapidly of the flushes, backache and vaginal irritation I had suffered for years. But it is awkward and embarrassing with my husband and children being registered with him.

If the individual doctor–patient relationship really breaks down the answer must be to change to someone else's list. But it is not so easy in busy urban areas to get on another list or to be sure you have not jumped out of the frying pan into the fire. The actual procedure is simple enough, and it does not necessarily involve you in embarrassing face-to-face contact with the doctor you are leaving. His secretary or receptionist will usually simply obtain his signature agreeing to the change on your medical card and hand this to you. This method should involve little delay, but the alternative of writing to the Executive Council for your area, explaining your reasons for wishing to change, means a twenty-one-day wait before you can apply to another doctor to be accepted. Before accepting you it is quite usual for the new doctor to ask to see you and perhaps just enquire why you are changing, but this can also give you a chance to find out his views on any matters of great importance to you, such as contraception or HRT, before committing yourself.

It has to be said that any partnership requires a degree of tact and patience on both sides, and women *demanding* a special form of treatment are likely to provoke resistance. Far better to ask gently to be considered for the treatment in a diplomatic manner, at least in the first instance, because your doctor rightly sees himself as the senior and professional partner. But all the same it is *your* body, *your* comfort, *your* health and in some situations *your* life which can be involved. This surely entitles you to some say.

We must not forget that while doctors may sometimes prescribe too much and listen too little, women may also demand too much and ask too little. Particularly where a drug new to them is being prescribed, a woman should always ask (if her doctors does not volunteer the information) what the drug is, what it does and what side-effects or risks could be involved.

But the key to this sort of two-way communication, which is the basis of good medicine, is time to talk, and under our present over-administered and under-funded NHS system, this is what is lacking. With its low level of per capita payments, doctors are forced to take on more patients than they should and are too hard-pressed to give an individual the time needed.

Under the present stringent economic circumstances, some doctors, such as Joe Jordan, believe more use should be made of less qualified and even non-medical people for much of the preliminary screening work. 'With special training this is already done very successfully in other countries,' he told me. 'I also believe we need more patient-education, leading to a degree of self-help for minor problems, so that doctors can give more time where and when it is really needed.'

If this book helps a little toward patient-education, or gives even a few women the courage and confidence to begin to really talk to their doctors and move toward a true doctor–patient partnership, it will have at least achieved something. If it can persuade women to fight for a properly funded Health Service with more emphasis on preventive medicine, it will be even more useful.

Medical references

1. Rayner, P. H. W., in *Problems of Childhood* (1976), British Medical Association, 131–8.
2. Knuth, Hull and Jacobs (1977), *British Journal of Obstetrics and Gynaecology 84*, 11: 801–7.
3. Hunter, D. J. S. (1977), *The Practioner 219*, 1312: 564–70.
4. Smith, T. C. G. (1978), *Pulse 36*, 4: 37.
   Cooper, W. (1978), *Modern Medicine 23*, No. 1, 53–5.
5. Dalton (1973), *Update 7*, 7: 833–9.
6. Dalton (1978), *Journal of Pharmacotherapy 1*, 2: 51–5.
7. Taylor, R. W. (1977), *Current Medical Research and Opinion 4*, Sup. 4, 35–40.
8. Brush, M. G. (1977), *Current Medical Research and Opinion 4*, Sup. 4, 9–15.
9. Giles, P. H. F. (personal communication to Professor R. W. Taylor).
10. Brush, M. G. (1977), *Current Medical Research and Opinion 4*, Sup. 4, 14.
11. Rosseinsky, D. R., and Hall, P. G., *Lancet 2*, 1024.
12. James, W. H. (1976), *Annals of Human Biology 3*, 6: 549–56.
13. Hurst, P. R., Eckstein, P., *et al.* (1977), *Nature 269*, 5626: 331–3.
14. Vessey, Martin (1976), summary in *Editorial Journal of Biosocial Science 8*, 4: 375–6.
15. Royal College of General Practitioners Report (1974), 22–30.
16. Vessey, McPherson and Johnson (1977), *Lancet 2*, 8041: 731–3.
    Royal College of General Practitioners (1977), *Lancet 2*, 8041: 727–31.
    Editorial (1977), *Lancet 2*, 8041: 747–8.
17. Kane, F. J. (1976), *American Journal of Obstetrics and Gynecology 126*, 968.
18. Winston, F. (1969), *Lancet 1*, 1209.
    Winston, F. (1969), *Lancet 2*, 877.
19. Adams, P. W. *et al.* (1973), *Lancet 1*, 898–904.
    Adams, P. W. *et al.* (1974), *Lancet 2*, 516–17.
    Wynne, V. (1975), *Lancet 1*, 561–4.

20. Goldzieher, J. A. and Green, J. A. (1962), *Journal of Clinical Endocrinology 22*, 325.
21. Mears, E. (1962), *British Medical Journal 2*, 75.
    Mears, E. (1965), *Handbook on Oral Contraception* (J. and A. Churchill, London).
22. Brewer, C. (1977), *British Medical Journal 1*, 476–7.
23. Hendry, Sommerville, Hall and Pugh (1973), *British Journal of Urology 41*, 684–92.
24. Logan-Edwards, R. (1964), *Proceedings of the Royal Society of Medicine 57*, No. 10, Part 1, 927–31 (section of Obstetrics and Gynaecology, 35–9).
    Crooke, A. C., Butt, W. R. *et al.* (1964), *Journal of Obstetrics and Gynaecology of the British Commonwealth 71*, 571–85.
25. Bromhall, J. D. (1975), *Nature 258*, 5537: 719–22.
26. Scrimjeour, J. B. (1978), *Toward Prevention of Foetal Malformation* (Edinburgh University Press).
27. Studd, J. W. W. (1973), *British Medical Journal 4*, 451.
28. Forest, A. P. M. (1974), in *The Treatment of Breast Cancer*, ed. Sir Hedley Atkins (M.T.P. Press, London), 9–48.
29. Strax, P. *et al.* (1970), *Archives of Environmental Health 20*, 758–63.
30. Fisher, B. *et al.* (1975), *New England Journal of Medicine 292*, 117–22.
    Bonadonna, G. *et al.* (1976), *New England Journal of Medicine 294*, 405–10.
31. Singer, Reid and Coppelson (1976), *American Journal of Obstetrics and Gynecology 126*, 1: 110–15.

Select bibliography

Bourne, Gordon. *Pregnancy.* Pan, 1975.

Cauthery, P., and Cole, M. *The Fundamentals of Sex.* W. H. Allen, 1971.

Comfort, Alex. *The Joy of Sex.* Quartet, 1974.

Dalton, Katherina. *Premenstrual Syndrome.* Heinemann, 1964.

Delvin, David. *The Book of Love.* New English Library, 1974.

Houghton, Peter and Elaine. *Unfocussed Grief.* The Birmingham Settlement, 1977.

Kilmartin, Angela. *Understanding Cystitis.* Pan, 1975.

Llewellyn-Jones, Derek. *Everywoman.* Faber, 1971.

— *Sex and V.D.* Faber, 1975.

Phillipp, Elliot. *Childlessness.* Arrow, 1976.

Rudinger, Edith, ed. *Infertility.* Consumers' Association, 1972.

— *The Newborn Baby.* Consumers' Association, 1973.

Advisory centres

Abortion

British Pregnancy Advisory Service
Austy Manor, Wootton Wawen
Solihull, West Midlands B95 6DA (head office)
(Henley-in-Arden 3225)
Also sterilization, pregnancy testing, low-cost vasectomy counselling and operations. Registered charity. Branches throughout the country.

Adoption and fostering

Adoption Resource Exchange
40 Brunswick Square, London WC1
(01-837 0496)
Specializes in trying to place older, handicapped or black children through adoption centres

Association of British Adoption and Fostering Agencies
4 Southampton Row, London WC1
(01-242 8951)
Represents most adoption, fostering and allied organizations. Gives general information and lists of adoption agencies in Britain

National Foster Care Association
80 Belmont Park, London SE13 5BN
(01-852 6821)
Co-ordinating body for 200 local groups. Provides information on problems of fostering, advising parents and those considering fostering

Anorexia

Anorexic Aid
Gravel House, Copthall Corner
Shalford St Peter, Bucks
(Gerrard's Cross 84844)
Support group with branches in major cities

Anorexics Anonymous
Mr J. Hevesi
24 Westmoreland Road
Barnes, London SW13
(01-748 4587)

Cancer

Women's National Cancer Control Campaign
1 South Audley St, London W1Y 5DQ
(01-499 7532/4)
Promotes measures for early detection and treatment of cervical and breast cancer: Provides leaflets, posters, films and breast-screening details; also runs mobile screening units

Mastectomy Association
Betty Westgate
1 Colworth Rd, Croydon, Surrey
(01-654 8643)
Help for mastectomy patients: self-help group; trained counselling by letter or telephone, booklets and visits, etc.

Childbirth

National Birthday Trust
57 Lower Belgrave St, London SW1
(01-730 5076)
Campaigns for extension and improvement of maternity services

Contraception

Area Health Authority clinics

Family Planning Association
27 Mortimer St, London W1N 7RJ
(01–636 7866)
Most family planning clinics are now run by AHAs but the FPA itself still runs about twenty clinics, offering in addition such services as advice on vasectomy and sub-fertility, and counselling on psycho-sexual problems

Brook Advisory Centres
233 Tottenham Court Rd, London W1 (head office)
(01–580 2991)
There are five centres in London and affiliated organizations in other cities

*(e.g. Coventry, Birmingham, Bristol, Cambridge, Liverpool and Edinburgh).
Caters particularly for birth control needs and sexual or emotional problems
of the unmarried*

Marie Stopes House
108 Whitfield St, London W1
(01–388 0622)
*Birth control services and information, pregnancy testing, female
sterilization and out-patient vasectomy*

Cystitis

The U and I Club
9E Compton Road, London N1
(01–730 5076)
Help and advice for cystitis sufferers

General aid or emergency help

Samaritans
17 Uxbridge Rd, Slough, Bucks.
(Slough 32713)
*Twenty-four-hour, confidential and free support service by telephone and in
person. Staffed by 19 000 volunteers in 167 branches nationwide.
See local phone book for addresses and numbers*

Release
1 Elgin Avenue, London W9
(01–289 1123 or 01–603 8654 in emergency)
*Advises and assists with legal problems, information on abuse of drugs –
mainly for young people*

Citizens' Advice Bureaux
26 Bedford Square, London WC1 (head office)
(01–636 4066)
*Has 710 bureaux nationally offering free information or referral to
specialist agencies; addresses from local phone books, town halls,
or from head office (above)*

Infertility

National Association for the Childless
The Birmingham Settlement
318 Summer Lane, Birmingham B19 3RL

One-parent families

National Council for One-Parent Families
255 Kentish Town Road, London NW5
(01–267 1361)
Information by letter, telephone or interview for single, separated, divorced or widowed parents from qualified social workers. Advice on pregnancy outside marriage and welfare benefits, etc.

Gingerbread
35 Wellington St, London WC2
(01–240 0953)
Has 330 local groups to help one-parent families

Pregnancy testing

British Pregnancy Advisory Service
Austy Manor, Wootton Wawen
Solihull, West Midlands B95 6DA (head office)
(Henley-in-Arden 3225)

Pregnancy Advisory Service
40 Margaret Street, London W1
(01–409 0281)

Ulster Pregnancy Advisory Association
338A Lisburn Rd, Belfast 9
(0232–667345)
Pregnancy testing and help if abortion is required

Vasectomy advice

Marie Stopes House
108 Whitfield St, London W1
(01–388 0622)
Low-cost vasectomy counselling and operations

Vasectomy, Crediton Project
West Longsight, Crediton, Devon
(Honiton 3165)
Provides both doctors and patients with information about vasectomy

Index